Medical Ethics

Saleh Abbas

Medical Ethics

Soft Skills for Clinical Care Providers

Springer

Saleh Abbas
Department of Surgery
Deakin University
Geelong, VIC, Australia

ISBN 978-981-96-9198-2 ISBN 978-981-96-9199-9 (eBook)
https://doi.org/10.1007/978-981-96-9199-9

This Springer imprint is published by the registered company Springer Nature Singapore Pte Ltd.
The registered company address is: 152 Beach Road, #21-01/04 Gateway East, Singapore 189721, Singapore

Preface

When I pursued my medical education in the 1980s, medicine was presented as a discipline grounded in extensive knowledge, rigorous scientific experimentation, refined artistry and accumulated experience. Occasionally, I would hear discussions about ethics and its pivotal role in clinical care, yet ethical principles were conspicuously absent from the curriculum. On the momentous day of our graduation in July 1987, the Dean of the medical school in Baghdad convened us in a grand lecture hall to recite the Hippocratic Oath. Most of my peers had only a vague understanding of the profound obligations the oath entailed, perceiving it instead as a testament to the personal integrity of the physician. I, too, was unaware of any texts dedicated to biomedical or clinical ethics, and the subject remained enigmatic throughout my early years in the field. In the 1990s, when I relocated to New Zealand, the landscape of clinical practice had notably evolved, and ethics had become a fundamental component in the curricula of numerous medical schools worldwide. This book is crafted to serve as a comprehensive reference for the myriad ethical challenges encountered by healthcare providers, ranging from medical students to seasoned physicians across all specialties, as well as nurses and administrative executives engaged in healthcare decision-making and service provision.

Medicine is more than a mere science—it is a profoundly human act. Every clinical skill performed at the bedside, every decision made in the consultation room, and every conversation held with patients embodies not only technical precision but also profound ethical responsibility.

This book emerged from the intricate intersection of two essential dimensions of medical practice: the mastery of clinical skills and the judicious application of biomedical ethics. While clinical competence guarantees that we are capable of acting, ethics ensures that we understand: when, how and why we should act.

Drawing from vivid real-world scenarios, cutting-edge debates and evidence-based practice, this text is meticulously crafted to equip current and future healthcare professionals with the tools necessary to navigate both the procedural and moral complexities of modern medicine. It strives to bridge the gap between technical proficiency and thoughtful consideration, between the quantifiable and the meaningful.

Whether you are a medical student embarking on the journey of taking a history for the first time, a seasoned clinician reflecting on ethical quandaries in daily practice or an educator inspiring deeper dialogue among learners, I hope this book provides clarity, challenge and compassion.

In an era where healthcare is increasingly influenced by technology, systems and external pressures, may we always remember the patient as a person—and the weighty responsibility we carry as healers.

Geelong, VIC, Australia Saleh Abbas

Introduction

Throughout history, various cultures and religions have emphasised the sanctity and dignity of human life. These beliefs have influenced modern Western medicine's ethical principles. In early civilisations like Egypt, Greece and Israel, there were ethical codes condemning the taking of human life. Judaism, for instance, introduced the idea that humans are created in the image of God, emphasising the sacredness of human life. Christianity and later Islam adopted similar beliefs.

When Christianity merged with Greco-Roman culture in the fourth century CE, these ideas spread throughout Western societies, including North America. Despite the separation of religion and government in Western countries, the moral teachings of Abrahamic religions still influence healthcare policies and ethical codes. Other cultures, like the Hippocratic physicians in polytheistic societies, also valued the sanctity of human life.

Modern debates in healthcare ethics focus on when human rights should be granted, especially regarding issues like embryonic development and end-of-life care. Scientific advancements have raised questions about the timing of when a human gains rights, and cases of patients regaining consciousness challenge the determination of when a soul departs the body.

The Declaration of Geneva and the International Code of Medical Ethics, drafted after World War II, initially protected the rights of the unborn but gradually removed such language. These ethical dilemmas require balancing core principles like beneficence, patient autonomy, non-maleficence and the sanctity of human life when making morally acceptable decisions.

The Oath of Hippocrates, which outlines fundamental principles for the behaviour of physicians, originates from the fifth century BCE. These principles safeguard the rights of patients and encourage physicians to act selflessly towards them on a voluntary basis. It underwent modifications in the tenth or eleventh century AD, removing references to pagan deities. The Oath is widely employed in various forms, serving as a guideline for aspiring medical professionals as they enter medical school or upon graduation [1].

In 1803, Thomas Percival, a British physician and philosopher, published a Code of Medical Ethics that delineated professional responsibilities and ideal conduct, particularly concerning hospitals and charitable institutions. During the inaugural meeting of the American Medical Association (AMA) in Philadelphia, PA, in 1847, two primary agenda items were the formulation of a code of ethics and the specification of minimum requirements for medical education and training. The Code of Ethics adopted at this meeting was greatly influenced by Percival's Medical Ethics [2, 3].

> The Hippocratic Oath (c. 400 BC) incorporates the obligations of non-maleficence and beneficence: "I will follow that system of regimen which, according to my ability and judgment, I consider for the benefit of my patients, and abstain from whatever is deleterious and mischievous". [1, 3]

American Medical Association Principles of Medical Ethics (1957)

These principles serve as guidelines to assist physicians, both individually and collectively, in upholding a high standard of ethical conduct. They are not legal statutes but rather standards against which a physician can assess the appropriateness of their actions in their interactions with patients, colleagues, allied professionals, and the general public.

Section 1: The primary objective of the medical profession is to provide service to humanity while fully respecting human dignity. Physicians should earn the trust of the patients under their care, offering each patient a comprehensive service.

Section 2: Physicians should continually strive to enhance their medical knowledge and skills, sharing the benefits of their professional expertise with both their patients and colleagues.

Section 3: Physicians should practice a healing method based on a solid scientific foundation and should avoid professional associations with individuals who undermine this principle.

Section 4: The medical profession must protect the public and itself from physicians who exhibit moral or professional deficiencies. Physicians should abide by all relevant laws, uphold the honour and integrity of the profession, and adhere to its self-imposed ethical standards. They should promptly report any illegal or unethical behaviour by fellow professionals without hesitation.

Section 5: Physicians have the autonomy to choose their patients, but they must provide emergency assistance to the best of their ability when needed. Once a physician has accepted a patient's care, they may not abandon the patient without adequate notice, unless formally discharged. Physicians should refrain from soliciting patients.

Section 6: Physicians should not engage in agreements that compromise their independent medical judgment, professional skills, or the quality of medical care.

Section 7: In their medical practice, physicians should derive their income solely from the provision of medical services, either directly by themselves or under their supervision, to their patients. Fees charged should be fair, considering the services provided and the patient's financial situation. Physicians should neither offer nor accept commissions for patient referrals. The dispensing of drugs, remedies, or medical devices is acceptable when it is in the best interests of the patient.

Section 8: Physicians should seek consultation when requested, especially in cases of uncertainty or complexity, or when it can enhance the quality of medical care.

Section 9: Physicians must maintain patient confidentiality and should not disclose information entrusted to them during medical care unless required by law or necessary to protect the individual or community's welfare.

Section 10: The ethical principles of the medical profession imply that physicians have responsibilities not only to individual patients but also to society as a whole. Physicians should actively engage in activities aimed at improving both individual and community health and well-being, reflecting the honoured ideals of the profession [4].

In 1803, English physician Thomas Percival published "Medical Ethics", a significant work that has successively inspired modern codes of medical ethics, including the inaugural edition of the American Medical Association's ethical guidelines in 1847. Despite its undeniable impact on the codification of medical ethics principles, scholars and experts hold diverse and conflicting perspectives on the true nature of this book. In the late eighteenth century, European urbanisation driven by the industrial revolution led to challenges for the migrating population into large cities, including diseases and poverty. Enlightenment ideals of tolerance fostered a rising commitment to assisting the lower classes. This support triggered the evolution of hospitals, transforming them into institutions focused on the social dimension of public health through a process of modernisation [5].

In 1789, Manchester faces a typhus epidemic that severely impacts the hospital's functionality. To address organisational challenges, the hospital managers decide to double the staff. However, the increased personnel leads to internal conflicts, the situation was messy and filled with perplexities. By 1791, with the epidemic ongoing, disputes escalate, resulting in the closure of the ward. In response to the scandal, the hospital appoints Thomas Percival, a prominent member, to develop a code of conduct aimed at disciplining staff behaviour, the title Medical Ethics was officially born in 1803, Thomas Gisborne used the definition of "applied moral philosophy" and David Hume analysed the notion of "practical morals" to distinguish it from more abstract speculations [6]. Therefore, Medical Ethics marked a clear departure from ancient Hippocratic ethics to establish the inaugural modern Code of medical ethics. Its principles have endured unchanged to the present day.

References

1. Council on Ethical and Judicial Affairs. Code of medical ethics – current opinions, 2002–2003 Edition. Chicago: American Medical Association; 2001.
2. Pellegrino ED. Thomas Percival's ethics: the ethics beneath the etiquette. In: Percival T, editor. Medical ethics. Birmingham: Classics of Medicine Library; 1985. p. 1–52.
3. Baker RB. The American medical ethics revolution. In: Baker RB, editor. The American medical ethics revolution. Baltimore: Johns Hopkins University Press; 1999. p. 17–51.
4. American Medical Association. Principles of medical ethics. Appendix F. In: Baker RB, editor. The American medical ethics revolution. Baltimore: Johns Hopkins University Press; 1957. p. 255–357.
5. Patuzzo S, Goracci G, Ciliberti R. Thomas Percival. Discussing the foundation of medical ethics. Acta Biomed. 2018;89(3):343–8. https://doi.org/10.23750/abm.v89i3.7050. PMID: 30333457; PMCID: PMC6502118.
6. Percival T. Medical ethics. Italian translation by Goracci Giada. In: Patuzzo S, editor. Milano: Mimesis; 2015. p. 11–30.

Contents

Chapter 1
Principles and Values

Autonomy

Respect for autonomy and respect for persons are closely intertwined, as it entails honouring the ideals, beliefs, and values of autonomous individuals. It signifies recognising the capacity and entitlement of individuals to make decisions about their own lives.

Beneficence

A principle of beneficence involves a normative statement that conveys a moral duty to act in a way that benefits others, assisting them in advancing their significant and lawful interests. This may involve averting or alleviating potential harm.

Capacity

Capacity entails the capability to provide informed consent for a specific treatment at a specific moment. A person possesses the capacity to provide informed consent for treatment or medical procedures if they: Comprehend the information provided to them regarding the treatment. Retain the pertinent information related to the decision. Evaluate or balance the relevant information essential to the decision. Effectively convey their decision [1].

S. Abbas, *Medical Ethics*, https://doi.org/10.1007/978-981-96-9199-9_1

Confidentiality

The statement, "The obligation not to disseminate patients' private information without their permission," underscores the fundamental principle of patient confidentiality within the healthcare profession. It signifies that healthcare professionals have a moral and legal responsibility to safeguard the personal and sensitive information shared by patients during the course of their medical care. Patient confidentiality is an ethical cornerstone, as it ensures that individuals can trust healthcare providers with their personal and medical histories without fear of unauthorised disclosure.

Moreover, when it is mentioned that "professionals are obligated to preserve confidential information to the extent permitted by good practice and the law," it implies that healthcare providers must adhere to established ethical norms and legal standards while maintaining patient confidentiality. This obligation suggests that professionals are responsible not only for respecting patients' privacy but also for staying well-informed about the evolving legal requirements and ethical guidelines governing patient information. They should act in accordance with these regulations and provide appropriate levels of data protection from unauthorised disclosure [2, 3].

Conscientious Objection

Conscientious objection in the medical context occurs when a doctor, due to a personal conflict with their own deeply-held beliefs or values, declines to offer or engage in a legal and justified treatment or procedure that aligns with established professional standards. It is crucial to emphasise that conscientious objection is rooted in genuine moral convictions and ethical concerns, rather than personal gain or discriminatory motives. In certain circumstances, it is considered ethically acceptable for a doctor to abstain from providing or participating in specific medical treatments or procedures based on their conscientious objection.

However, it is vital to recognise that a doctor's decision to abstain from providing or participating in a treatment or procedure due to conscientious objection has a direct impact on patients. Therefore, doctors bear an ethical responsibility to minimise any disruptions to patient care resulting from their objection. They should never exploit conscientious objection as a means to deliberately obstruct patients' access to necessary healthcare services. This underscores the delicate balance that healthcare professionals must strike between their own beliefs and their commitment to providing the best possible care for their patients [1, 2].

Deontological Ethics

Deontological ethics is a normative ethical theory that posits the right course of action as one that aligns with a universal rule, duty, or moral law that can be universally applied.

Immanuel Kant's concept of "The categorical imperative" underscores the principle that individuals should act in a manner that would be morally acceptable if everyone were to act in the same way. Moreover, it emphasises the importance of not treating individuals solely as a means to an end, where the outcome is the sole consideration [1].

Equality

Equality asserts that every human being is inherently born free and equal, grounded in the idea that all individuals possess identical rights and merit equal respect. It underscores the entitlement of every person to fair and impartial treatment."

Bioethics

Bioethics is a field of practical ethics that explores three primary subfields: medical ethics, animal rights, and environmental ethics. While each of these subfields primarily concerns itself with different subjects—namely, humans, animals, and the environment—there exists a substantial overlap in terms of specific issues, fundamental principles, theories, and prominent lines of reasoning.

Equity

The notion of equity pertains to the "elimination of unnecessary, unjust, or correctable disparities among various groups of people, whether such groups are defined socially, economically, demographically, geographically, or through other stratifying methods [4].

Honesty and Truthfulness

The medical profession's acknowledgment of the shift from paternalism to respecting patient autonomy underscores the obligation for doctors to be honest, as patients anticipate truthfulness from their physicians.

Informed Consent

Informed consent is typically a process in which healthcare professionals offer information to patients and assist them in comprehending the information, enabling patients to decide whether to accept or decline treatment in alignment with their values [1].

Justice

Justice entails the assessment of how benefits and burdens are allocated within a society. Various forms of justice exist, including distributive, procedural, social, and retributive justice. Nevertheless, distributive justice holds particular relevance in the realm of healthcare [1].

Narrative Ethics

A normative ethical perspective, emphasising the significance of personal narratives in ethical analysis and decision-making, acknowledges the influence of personal, social, and cultural elements. Its objective is to gain insight into the subjective meanings of a situation to those involved, facilitating the pursuit of an ethical resolution [5].

Non-maleficence

"The obligation to avoid harm," The principle of non-maleficence entails the duty to avoid imposing risks of harm and to refrain from causing actual harm. This raises the question of whether the principle of non-maleficence has been breached in clinical scenarios where it can be objectively determined that the potential risks of a recommended treatment, whether it's a procedure or medication, outweigh the anticipated benefits, taking all factors into account [1, 3].

Privacy

Privacy delineates a boundary within which we regulate the access to information concerning ourselves. The definition of privacy is challenging due to its encompassing various domains, including information privacy, bodily privacy, privacy of communications, and territorial privacy [1, 3].

Public Health Ethics

Public health ethics primarily explores the moral principles and rationales behind public health initiatives, ethical dilemmas arising from resource constraints in health promotion, and potential conflicts between communal well-being and personal freedoms. As an academic discipline, public health ethics aims to elucidate the guiding principles and values underpinning public health practices. These principles and values serve as a decision-making framework and a justification for the choices made [6].

Reciprocity

"Reciprocity entails the exchange of resources or benefits between individuals or groups, where each party provides or allows something for the other's benefit."

In the doctor-patient relationship, mutual recognition is fostered. Both parties gain insights about each other, enabling one another while gaining self-awareness. Through the attentive practice of medicine, patients not only discover their biological conditions but also explore their emotional concerns and strengths. Simultaneously, physicians find their own reflections in the patient's perspective, leading to contemplation of their own values and priorities [7].

Respect for Human Dignity

The concept of human dignity encompasses the inherent worth of individuals who possess the capacities for reflection, sensitivity, verbal communication, free choice, self-determination, and creativity, at least potentially or as members of a natural kind.

Human dignity is a fundamental concept, and it is both theoretically and normatively inappropriate to reduce it to the functional characteristics of a person's abilities or autonomy. Respecting human dignity involves recognising the intrinsic worth of every human being."

"The perspective that individuals hold inherent value significantly influences everyday medical practice and can greatly enhance the doctor-patient relationship. Specifically, this outlook serves as a reminder to healthcare professionals that every patient, regardless of their diagnosis, is not merely a 'case,' 'disease,' or 'room number,' but a person deserving the utmost respect and care [8].

Utilitarianism

Utilitarianism stands out as one of the most influential and compelling normative ethical philosophies throughout the history of philosophy. Although various interpretations of this philosophy exist, the core idea of utilitarianism centres on the belief that the morally right action is the one that generates the greatest overall good for everyone involved. According to the utilitarian perspective, it is incumbent upon individuals to maximise the collective welfare, taking into account the well-being of others alongside their own. In its contemporary form, utilitarianism assesses actions based on their capacity to best fulfil the needs of all those impacted by the proposed action. This evaluation centres on the consequences and effects of actions, rather than the motives or intentions of the actor [3].

Values

Values represent what is significant and deserving of esteem, forming the foundation for moral principles and ethical contemplation. Everyone possesses their own values, influenced by various factors such as family, religion, peers, culture, ethnicity, social upbringing, gender, and more. Values play an instructive role for individuals, vocations, communities, and organisations. Values can be recognised across diverse cultures and populations... One of the primary objectives of ethics is to engage in intellectual examination of values and the conflicts that may arise, with the aim of delineating our ethical responsibilities [9].

Virtues

A virtue represents a personal characteristic or tendency that reflects an individual's commitment to a particular ethical value. Virtue ethics underscores the importance of fostering good character as the foundation for making virtuous choices and sound moral judgment [1].

Vulnerability

"When we fall ill, we become acutely aware of how our physical existence exposes us to unforeseen circumstances that can disrupt our daily activities and life's objectives. This experience may leave us feeling that our sense of freedom is diminished, and our life's opportunities are altered."

"Human suffering and distress are reflections of our inherent vulnerability. They present us with a dual challenge: we must work to minimise suffering while also acknowledging it as an inherent aspect of life. Human vulnerability should not be viewed merely as an adversary to be eradicated."

When utilising and advancing scientific knowledge, medical practices, and related technologies, it is essential to consider human vulnerability. We must take into account the special vulnerability of certain individuals and groups, ensuring their protection and respecting the personal integrity of those affected [9].

References

1. Jones GE, DeMarco JP. Bioethics in context: moral, legal and social perspectives. Ontario, Canada: Broadview Press; 2016.
2. Chowning JT, Fraser P. An ethics primer. Seattle WA: Northwest Association of Biomedical Research; 2007.
3. Breen KJ, Cordner SM, Thomson CJH, Plueckhahn VD. Good medical practice: professionalism, ethics and law. New York: Cambridge University Press; 2010.
4. United Nations Educational, Scientific and Cultural Organisation (UNESCO). Sector for Social and Human Sciences: Division of Ethics of Science and Technology; 2016. Bioethics Core Curriculum, Section 1: Syllabus Ethics Education Program.
5. Tovey P. Narrative and knowledge development in medical ethics. J Med Ethics. 1998;24:176.
6. Faden R, Shebaya S. Public health ethics. In: Zalta EN, editor. The Stanford encyclopedia of philosophy; 2016.
7. Charon R. The reciprocity of recognition—what medicine exposes about self and other. N Engl J Med. 2012;367(20):1878.
8. Andorno R. Human dignity and human rights as a common ground for a global bioethics. J Med Philos. 2009;34:223.
9. United Nations Educational, Scientific and Cultural Organisation (UNESCO). Universal Declaration on Bioethics and Human Rights; 2006. Available from: https://unesdoc.unesco.org/ark:/48223/pf0000146180.

Chapter 2
Philosophical Background of Medical Ethics

Americans have a tendency to believe that when there's a problem there must be a solution.

—Henry Kissinger

Ethics is an intrinsic and inextricable element of clinical medicine. As physicians, we shoulder an ethical obligation to (i) foster the patient's well-being, (ii) mitigate or avert harm, and (iii) respect the patient's values and preferences. We must consistently persevere to perform to the utmost of our abilities for our patients, regardless of the circumstances or repercussions.

Indeed, it is remarkably challenging for those of us in the twenty-first century, with our access to cutting-edge modern medicine and healthcare, to fully grasp how humanity endured in the past without these medical advancements. The evolution of medicine over the centuries has profoundly enhanced our quality of life, significantly extended our lifespans, and offered resolutions to myriad ailments and health obstacles. Nonetheless, it is crucial to acknowledge and cherish the contributions of our predecessors in the medical field and their varied methodologies, which formed the bedrock for the astounding achievements we enjoy today. The history of medicine stands as a powerful testament to human ingenuity, innovation, and tenacity in confronting health adversities.

While the evolution of medicine has undeniably ushered in substantial advancements in healthcare and elevated the overall quality of life for countless individuals, it is equally true that certain facets of contemporary medicine can carry unforeseen consequences.

Side Effects

Many medications and medical treatments carry potential side effects and risks. In some cases, the cure or treatment can result in new health issues or complications.

S. Abbas, *Medical Ethics*, https://doi.org/10.1007/978-981-95-9199-9_2

Overmedicalisation

The overuse or misuse of medical interventions, such as unnecessary surgeries or excessive prescription of medications, can lead to complications and adverse outcomes.

Antibiotic Resistance

The widespread use of antibiotics has led to the development of antibiotic-resistant bacteria, posing a significant threat to public health.

Technological Errors

As medical technology becomes more complex, the potential for errors in diagnosis or treatment increases, which can have serious consequences.

Health Inequality

Access to advanced medical care is unevenly distributed, leading to disparities in health outcomes. Some individuals may not have access to the benefits of modern medicine.

Ethical Dilemmas

Advances in medical technology often raise complex ethical questions, such as those related to end-of-life care, genetic manipulation, and the use of emerging technologies like artificial intelligence in healthcare decision-making.

Environmental Impact

The production and disposal of medical equipment and pharmaceuticals can have environmental impacts, contributing to pollution and waste.

It is important to recognise that while modern medicine has brought about numerous benefits, it also requires careful consideration of its ethical, social, and environmental implications. Striking a balance between medical progress and ensuring the well-being of individuals and society as a whole is an ongoing challenge in the field of medicine.

The precise count of fatalities resulting from medical errors in the United States can be remarkably difficult to ascertain with exactitude. Estimations of yearly mortalities attributable to medical errors depend on a multitude of studies and data sources, which naturally lead to a range of figures. Nonetheless, it is broadly acknowledged that medical errors stand as a substantial cause of death in the United States. A commonly referenced assessment originates from a 2013 study published in the *Journal of Patient Safety*, which posited that medical errors might account for between 210,000 and 440,000 fatalities each year in American hospitals. While this estimate serves as a pivotal reference, it is crucial to acknowledge that varying studies and methodologies can produce somewhat divergent results.

Moreover, it is vital to understand that medical errors span a wide array of concerns, including misdiagnoses, medication errors, surgical lapses, and communication failings. The healthcare sector continues to strive relentlessly to mitigate medical errors and enhance patient safety in response to this pressing issue.

It is fitting to credit the codification of medical ethics to Hippocrates, the esteemed ancient Greek physician who is frequently hailed as the "Father of Medicine." Living approximately between 460 and 370 BCE, Hippocrates is celebrated for his profound contributions to medical knowledge, practice, and ethical standards. He is most celebrated for the "Hippocratic Oath," a revered vow that practitioners of medicine customarily swear upon joining the profession. This oath delineates a set of ethical principles and directives for physicians, encompassing pledges to:

Beneficence

The oath requires physicians to act in the best interests of their patients, prioritising their well-being and health.

Nonmaleficence

Physicians promise to do no harm, avoiding actions that could harm patients intentionally.

Patient Confidentiality

The oath stresses the importance of keeping patients' medical information confidential, and respecting their privacy.

Informed Consent

Physicians pledge to inform patients fully about their medical conditions, treatment options, and potential risks so that patients can make informed decisions about their care.

Professional Integrity

The oath emphasises the need for honesty, integrity, and professionalism in medical practice.

While the Hippocratic Oath is a foundational document in the history of medical ethics, it is essential to recognise that ethical considerations in medicine existed before Hippocrates. Various ancient cultures, such as the Egyptians and Babylonians, had their codes of medical ethics and moral guidelines for physicians. However, Hippocrates' contributions are significant because they marked a formal and systematic approach to ethics in medicine that has had a lasting influence on Western medical ethics and the principles of medical professionalism.

In summary, while medical ethics existed in various forms in different cultures before Hippocrates, he is credited with formalising and codifying many of the ethical principles that continue to guide medical practice today.

Modern medical ethics as a distinct academic and ethical discipline began to take shape in the mid-twentieth century. It emerged in response to complex ethical dilemmas posed by advances in medicine, technology, and healthcare delivery. Several key developments and events contributed to the establishment of modern medical ethics:

Nuremberg Code (1947)

In the aftermath of World War II, the Nuremberg Trials addressed the unethical medical experiments conducted by Nazi doctors. The Nuremberg Code, developed during these trials, laid down principles for ethical human experimentation, emphasising the importance of informed consent and the well-being of research subjects.

Declaration of Helsinki (1964)

The World Medical Association introduced the Declaration of Helsinki, which provided ethical guidelines for medical research involving human subjects. It has undergone several revisions and remains a crucial document in the field of medical ethics.

Belmont Report (1979)

In the United States, the Belmont Report was issued by the National Commission for the Protection of Human Subjects of Biomedical and Behavioural Research. It established principles for ethical research involving human subjects, emphasising respect for persons, beneficence, and justice.

Bioethics and Medical Humanities

The 1960s and 1970s witnessed the emergence of bioethics as an academic discipline, with significant contributions from scholars such as Joseph Fletcher, Tom L Beauchamp, and James Childress. Bioethics integrated ethical considerations into various aspects of healthcare, including medical research, clinical practice, and healthcare policy. Additionally, medical humanities programs started to examine the ethical, social, and cultural dimensions of medicine

Establishment of Ethics Committees: Many healthcare institutions started establishing ethics committees to address ethical issues in clinical care, research, and policy. These committees played a pivotal role in shaping ethical practices within healthcare settings.

Medical Ethics Journals: The publication of dedicated medical ethics journals, such as the Journal of Medical Ethics (established in 1975), provided a platform for scholars to disseminate research and engage in ethical discourse.

Legislation and Regulation

Governments and healthcare organisations across the globe commenced the implementation of laws, regulations, and guidelines that underscored ethical considerations in healthcare, such as the rights of patients, informed consent, and policies for organ transplantation.

Modern medical ethics is a vibrant and ever-evolving domain, adeptly adapting to the myriad challenges presented by medical innovations, shifts in cultural norms, and the changing expectations of society. This field encompasses a broad spectrum of issues, including end-of-life care, the allocation of resources, genetic and reproductive ethics, research ethics, and the ethical application of emerging technologies in healthcare. As a scholarly discipline, it serves a crucial function in steering ethical decision-making within the realms of medical practice and biomedical research.

Medical schools typically include medical ethics as an integral part of their curriculum, and the teaching of medical ethics is considered essential for several reasons.

Patient Welfare

Medical ethics education underscores the paramount importance of patient welfare and fervently encourages healthcare professionals to place the well-being of their patients at the forefront of their practice. It furnishes aspiring physicians with the profound knowledge and essential skills necessary to navigate and make sound ethical decisions that steadfastly advance the best interests of their patients. Certain medical institutions boast comprehensive medical humanities programs that meticulously examine the intricate ethical, cultural, and societal dimensions of medicine. These enriching programs delve into the profound interplay between medicine and disciplines such as literature, philosophy, and the arts.

Informed Consent

Understanding medical ethics is crucial for obtaining informed consent from patients. Healthcare providers must ensure that patients fully comprehend their medical conditions, treatment options, and potential risks, allowing them to make informed decisions about their care.

Ethical Dilemmas

Healthcare professionals often encounter complex ethical dilemmas in clinical practice. Teaching medical ethics helps students recognise and navigate these dilemmas, ensuring that ethical considerations are integrated into clinical decision-making. Ethics is often integrated into the teaching of clinical cases. Medical students learn not only the medical aspects of cases but also the ethical considerations involved in patient care.

Professionalism

Medical ethics is intricately intertwined with medical professionalism, instilling in students the essential values, attitudes, and behaviors that are anticipated of healthcare professionals, such as unwavering honesty, profound integrity, and a deep respect for the rights of patients.

End-of-Life Care

Medical ethics education prepares students to address sensitive issues related to end-of-life care, including decisions about withholding or withdrawing treatment, advance directives, and palliative care.

Research Ethics

Understanding research ethics is essential for medical students who may engage in clinical research. Ethical research practices protect the rights and well-being of research subjects and ensure the integrity of scientific inquiry.

Legal and Regulatory Compliance

Knowledge of medical ethics helps healthcare professionals comply with legal and regulatory requirements, such as those related to patient confidentiality and privacy.

Patient–Physician Communication

Effective communication with patients, including the thoughtful discussion of challenging topics and the delicate delivery of distressing news, is a crucial element of medical ethics education.

Cultural Competence

Medical ethics education fosters cultural competence by promoting a deep understanding of the diverse cultural beliefs and values and religions that significantly influence healthcare decisions. While medical ethics is an essential part of medical education, the extent and scope of ethics instruction can vary widely among medical schools. Some institutions integrate ethics into various courses throughout the curriculum, while others offer specialised ethics courses or seminars. Ethical case discussions, clinical ethics consultations, and interactions with ethics committees may also be integral components of the educational experience.

Philosophy plays a crucial role in shaping and understanding the foundations of medical ethics. Medical ethics refers to the moral principles and values that guide healthcare professionals in making decisions about patient care, treatment options, and research practices. Philosophy contributes to medical ethics in several ways.

Ethical Theories

Philosophy provides a sophisticated framework for understanding and evaluating a myriad of ethical theories that guide medical decision-making. For instance, utilitarianism, deontology, virtue ethics, and principlism are prominent ethical theories that help healthcare professionals carefully dissect complex ethical challenges and make thoroughly informed decisions.

Critical Thinking

Philosophy encourages critical thinking and logical reasoning, essential skills for healthcare professionals when they encounter ethical challenges. Philosophical analysis helps in identifying and clarifying the underlying values, principles, and assumptions that influence medical decisions.

Moral Reasoning

Medical ethics often involves navigating conflicting moral values and priorities. Philosophical tools aid in developing robust moral reasoning skills, enabling healthcare professionals to weigh the pros and cons of various courses of action and make ethically defensible choices.

Bioethical Issues

Most medical ethical dilemmas encompass intricate questions pertaining to the inception and conclusion of life, personal autonomy, informed consent, equitable justice, and the judicious distribution of scarce healthcare resources. Philosophical inquiry offers a robust framework for engaging with these subjects in a profound manner, nurturing a more nuanced comprehension of the moral dimensions underlying medical practices.

Religious Diversity

In a multicultural and diverse world, medical ethics must consider the varied cultural and religious perspectives on health and. Philosophical analysis allows for a respectful examination of these perspectives and aids in finding common ethical ground.

Ethical Dilemmas

Medicine frequently presents situations where ethical principles conflict. Philosophical reasoning offers a structured approach to address these dilemmas, helping healthcare professionals weigh competing values and arrive at ethically sound decisions.

Policy and Regulation

Philosophical thinking is instrumental in shaping healthcare policies and regulations. It helps in formulating guidelines that ensure patient rights, research ethics, and fair allocation of medical resources.

Patient–Physician Relationship

Philosophy contributes to understanding the ethical dimensions of the patient-physician relationship, emphasising trust, empathy, informed consent, and shared decision-making. These values are crucial for upholding patient dignity and autonomy.

Medical Research Ethics

Philosophical principles underpin the ethical conduct of medical research involving human subjects. Concepts like informed consent, beneficence, and respect for persons guide the development of ethical guidelines for research.

Continuing Ethical Discussions

Philosophy fosters ongoing discussions about the evolving ethical challenges posed by advances in medical technology, genetics, and other scientific fields. These discussions are essential for adapting ethical norms to changing circumstances.

In summary, philosophy provides the intellectual tools and frameworks necessary for healthcare professionals to navigate the intricate landscape of medical ethics. It equips them with the skills to analyse, reason, and make ethical decisions that prioritise patient well-being, respect for autonomy, and the principles of justice.

Several ethical theories serve as frameworks for addressing moral dilemmas in the field of medical ethics. These theories offer different perspectives on how to determine the right course of action when faced with complex medical decisions. Some of the prominent theories include:

Utilitarianism

Utilitarianism posits that the morally correct action is the one that maximises overall happiness or utility. In a medical setting, this theory would entail selecting the option that yields the most comprehensive well-being for the patients concerned. However, detractors contend that utilitarianism could easily neglect individual rights and may result in the sacrifice of the interests of a minority for the broader benefit.

Deontology

Deontological ethics focuses on following moral rules and duties, even if the results are not the best. In medicine, this means respecting patient choices, keeping their information private, and following rules like "do no harm" and "be honest." This approach values the dignity and rights of each person.

Virtue Ethics

Virtue ethics centres on cultivating virtuous character traits and moral virtues. In the context of medical ethics, healthcare professionals are encouraged to develop virtues like compassion, empathy, and integrity. This approach focuses on the long-term development of ethical individuals who consistently make virtuous choices.

Principlism

Principlism is a way to make decisions using key ethical rules. The four main rules are: respecting the patient's choices, helping the patient's well-being, avoiding harm, and being fair with resources and treatment. This method helps people analyse tough ethical problems.

Casuistry

Casuistry involves analysing specific cases and comparing them to similar cases from the past to derive ethical guidelines. In medical ethics, this approach relies on precedent and context to determine the morally appropriate action. It seeks to find relevant parallels between cases to guide decision-making.

Feminist Ethics

Feminist ethics highlights the importance of relational ethics, empathy, and context. It critiques traditional ethical theories for their lack of attention to issues such as gender bias, power dynamics, and care ethics. In medical ethics, a feminist perspective can shed light on the impact of social roles, inequalities, and caring relationships on healthcare decisions.

Narrative Ethics

Narrative ethics emphasises the significance of personal stories and experiences in ethical decision-making. It encourages understanding the narratives of patients, healthcare providers, and families to better appreciate the complexity of medical situations and the moral dimensions involved.

Cultural Relativism

This idea says that what is right and wrong is decided by each culture and can be different in different places. In medical ethics, it is important to respect different cultural rules while also thinking about basic human rights.

Ethics of Care

The ethics of care emphasises empathy, compassion, and the importance of relationships in moral decision-making. It critiques traditional ethical theories for their emphasis on abstract principles and instead focuses on the immediate needs and relationships of individuals involved.

These theories offer different lenses through which to examine medical ethical dilemmas. Often, real-world medical situations are complex and may require a combination of these theories or a customised approach that takes into account the unique circumstances of the case. Medical professionals and ethicists often engage in ongoing discussions to determine the most appropriate ethical framework for specific situations.

The philosophy of medicine is a branch of philosophy that examines the fundamental concepts, principles, and ethical issues related to the practice of medicine. It delves into questions about the nature of health and disease, the goals and values of medicine, the relationship between science and medicine, and the ethical considerations surrounding medical practices. Here are some key aspects of the philosophy of medicine:

Nature of Health and Disease

Philosophers of medicine explore the definitions of health and disease, considering whether these concepts are objective, culturally relative, or context-dependent. They analyse the distinction between normal functioning and pathological conditions, and they question whether there are universal criteria for determining what constitutes a disease.

Biopsychosocial Model

The philosophy of medicine often engages with the biopsychosocial model, which views health as the result of interactions among biological, psychological, and social factors. This holistic approach challenges reductionist views that focus solely on biological explanations for health and disease.

Medical Epistemology

This part looks at how healthcare professionals learn, use, and share medical knowledge. It talks about the link between evidence-based medicine and clinical judgment, how clinical experience plays a role, and how medical research affects the practical daily delivery of medical care.

Placebo Effect and Mind–Body Interaction

Philosophers of medicine delve into the intricate role of placebo effects and the nuanced mind–body interactions in medical treatments. They meticulously examine how patients' beliefs and expectations subtly influence treatment outcomes and thoughtfully consider the ethical ramifications of incorporating placebos in medical practice.

Medical Ethics

The philosophy of medicine intricately engages with the nuanced field of medical ethics, addressing pivotal issues such as meticulously informed consent, robust patient autonomy, compassionate end-of-life care, the equitable allocation of medical resources, ethically conducted experimentation on human subjects, and the dynamic relationship between healthcare professionals and their patients.

Pain and Suffering

Philosophers examine the nature of pain and suffering and explore ethical questions related to pain management, palliative care, and the relief of suffering in medical contexts.

Biotechnology and Enhancement

With advances in biotechnology, philosophers of medicine consider the ethical implications of medical interventions aimed at enhancing human capabilities beyond treating diseases. This includes discussions about cosmetic surgery, cognitive enhancers, and genetic engineering.

Public Health Ethics

This domain meticulously explores the intricate ethical considerations intertwined with public health policies, encompassing vital issues such as disease prevention, vaccination, quarantine, and the delicate equilibrium between individual freedoms and the overarching well-being of the community.

Existential and Phenomenological Perspectives

Some philosophers approach medicine from existential and phenomenological perspectives, exploring how illness, suffering, and mortality impact individuals' lived experiences and sense of self.

Medical Ontology

Medical ontology meticulously explores the intrinsic nature of medical entities, including diseases, treatments, and various medical conditions. It delves into nuanced questions regarding the ontological status of these entities and their intricate relationships with one another.

Narrative Medicine

This approach highlights the profound importance of delving into patients' personal narratives and experiences within medical practice. It emphasises the significance of attentively listening to patients' stories to offer more comprehensive and genuinely patient-centred care.

Professionalism and Virtue in Medicine

Philosophers explore the virtues and ethical standards that healthcare professionals should cultivate to ensure patient-centred care, trustworthiness, and professionalism.

Overall, the philosophy of medicine elegantly bridges the gap between the scientific, ethical, and humanistic dimensions of medical practice. It encourages profound reflection on the fundamental questions that underpin medical practice and assists healthcare professionals in navigating the intricate moral, epistemological, and ontological challenges they face in their work.

The trolley problem is a renowned thought experiment in ethics and philosophy that presents a morally complex dilemma involving a runaway trolley hurtling toward a group of individuals. The decision-maker is confronted with the agonising choice of either allowing the trolley to continue its inexorable course and harm multiple people or diverting it onto an alternative track to harm fewer individuals. This scenario provocatively raises questions about the morality of actively causing harm to save more lives versus refraining from intervention and allowing harm to transpire. While the trolley problem is frequently discussed within a broad ethical framework, it has also been applied to diverse fields, including the realm of medical ethics.

In the realm of medical ethics, the trolley problem can be ingeniously adapted to reflect the harrowing decisions that healthcare professionals might confront, especially in dire circumstances where the prioritisation of patient welfare is paramount. Consider this illustrative scenario within a bustling hospital: five patients, each gravely ill and in urgent need of distinct organ transplants (heart, lungs, liver, kidney, and pancreas), will almost certainly perish within a brief timeframe without intervention. Coincidentally, a robust individual, whose blood type matches the patients, is admitted for a routine examination. The medical team is then ensnared in a formidable ethical quandary: should they allow the five patients to succumb to their fates due to the scarcity of organs, or should they undertake the ethically fraught action of extracting organs from the healthy individual to preserve the lives of the five?

This nuanced medical ethics adaptation of the trolley problem places healthcare professionals in a position where they must confront the profound implications of actively inflicting harm (organ harvesting) to salvage multiple lives. The scenario fervently probes the tenets of beneficence (the pursuit of maximising patient benefits) and non-maleficence (the duty to prevent harm) within the medical domain. It also compels healthcare practitioners to grapple with the intricate equilibrium between the rights of individual patients and the pursuit of collective welfare.

The trolley problem in the medical context illustrates the complexity of ethical decision-making, where there are no easy answers and various ethical theories may lead to different conclusions. It encourages healthcare professionals to reflect on their moral values, ethical principles, and the potential consequences of their actions.

It is important to note that the trolley problem is a simplified thought experiment and does not encompass the full complexity of real-world medical situations. Medical ethics often involves multiple factors, uncertainties, and emotional considerations that go beyond the simple binary choices presented in the classic trolley problem. Nevertheless, using such thought experiments can help stimulate ethical discussions and encourage critical thinking about the moral dimensions of medical decisions. This book seeks to provide an in-depth understanding of explanation, causation, and experimentation, as well as debates over their applications in science. It will provide a comprehensive overview of the philosophical and scientific debates surrounding these topics, as well as suggestions for applications in the fields of biology, chemistry, physics, and psychology.

Further Readings

1. Steven H. Miles, the hippocratic oath and the ethics of medicine (New York: Oxford University Press, 2004), XIV + 208 pages. HEC Forum. 2005;17:237–9.
2. Beauchamp TL, Childress JF. Principles of biomedical ethics. Oxford University Press; 2019.
3. Storer I, Swartwood J. Doing practical ethics. Oxfors University Press; 2021.
4. Churchill LR. Ethics for everyone. Oxford University Press; 2020.
5. Thompson M. Ethics for life, teach yourself; 2018.

Chapter 3
Philosophy of Medicine

Philosophy of medicine explores key issues in the health sciences, such as metaphysics and epistemology. The field dates back to ancient times, but scholars have discussed key concepts since the 1800s. In the past, debates have occurred over whether or not there is a distinct field of medicine that can be termed "philosophy of medicine" (e.g., Caplan 1992). Caplan calls medical ethics, bioethics, health policy, and medical aesthetics examples of philosophy and medicine, but he sees the philosophy of medicine to be something quite different. He gives a comprehensive definition of philosophy of medicine, and explains why he believes it is an important and unique area of study: "The philosophy of medicine is the study of epistemological, metaphysical and methodological dimensions of medicine; therapeutic and experimental; diagnostic, therapeutic, and palliative." In his conclusion Caplan says "The philosophy of medicine as it currently exists fails to satisfy these criteria and, thus, fails to exist as a field of inquiry. The non-existence of the philosophy of medicine is unfortunate. Medicine and philosophy would both benefit from the development of the philosophy of medicine as a field" [1]. But many decades later we see the philosophy of medicine as a well established field with many journals dedicated to studying this field. Philosophy of science relied on philosophy of medicine in its journey for maturation.

Medicine indeed has a long history that predates the ancient Greeks, with significant contributions from civilisations such as the Babylonians, Egyptians, and others. What set the Greeks apart was their approach to medicine, which integrated philosophical thinking and systematic inquiry into the practice of medicine. Here are some key elements that highlight the Greek contribution:

S. Abbas, *Medical Ethics*, https://doi.org/10.1007/978-981-96-9199-9_3

Philosophical Inquiry

Greek philosophers, including figures like Hippocrates, Galen, and Aristotle, sought to understand the natural world and the human body through systematic observation and reasoning. This philosophical approach laid the groundwork for scientific inquiry in medicine.

Empirical Observation

Greek physicians emphasised the importance of empirical observation and clinical examination. They focused on gathering data, documenting symptoms, and making careful observations of patients' conditions.

Ethical Foundations

The Hippocratic Oath, attributed to Hippocrates, emphasised ethical principles in medical practice. This included commitments to patient confidentiality, informed consent, and the principle of "do no harm" (non-maleficence).

Naturalistic Explanations

Greek physicians moved away from supernatural and mystical explanations for diseases and instead sought naturalistic explanations rooted in anatomy, physiology, and the understanding of bodily functions.

Anatomy and Dissection

Greek physicians, particularly Herophilus and Erasistratus in Alexandria, made significant advancements in human anatomy through dissections of human cadavers. This empirical approach to understanding anatomy had a profound impact on medical knowledge.

Medical Treatises

Prominent Greek physicians authored medical treatises and texts that synthesised medical knowledge, making it accessible to others. These writings became foundational texts in the study and practice of medicine.

Teaching and Mentorship

Greek medical schools, such as the one in Alexandria, played a crucial role in the transmission of medical knowledge. They provided a structured education for aspiring physicians.

The fusion of philosophy, empirical observation, ethics, and systematic thinking in Greek medicine marked a significant departure from earlier medical traditions. While other civilisations had made important contributions to medicine, the Greeks laid the groundwork for a more scientific and rational approach to healthcare that has continued to evolve and shape modern medicine [2].

I swear by Apollo Physician and Asclepius and Hygieia and Panaceia and all the gods and goddesses, making them my witness, that I will fulfil according to my ability and judgment this oath and this covenant:

To hold him who has taught me this art as equal to my parents and to live my life in partnership with him, and if he is in need of money to give him a share of mine, and to regard his offspring as equal to my brothers in male lineage and to teach them this art-if they desire to learn it-without fee and covenant; to give a share of precepts and oral instruction and all the other learning to my sons and to the sons of him who has instructed me and to pupils who have signed the covenant and have taken an oath according to the medical law, but to no one else.

I will apply dietetic measures for the benefit of the sick according to my ability and judgment; I will keep them from harm and injustice.

I will neither give a deadly drug to anybody if asked for it nor will I make a suggestion to this effect. Similarly, I will not give to a woman an abortive remedy. In purity and holiness, I will guard my life and my art.

I will not use the knife, nor even on sufferers from stone, but will withdraw in favour of such men as are engaged in this work.

Whatever house I may visit, I will come for the benefit of the sick, remaining free of all intentional injustice, of all mischief and in particular sexual relations with both female and male persons, be they free or slaves.

Whatever I may see or hear in the course of the treatment in regard to the life of men, which on no account one must spread abroad, I will keep to myself holding such things shameful to be spoken about.

If I fulfil this oath and do not violate it, may it be granted to me to enjoy life and art, being honoured with fame among all men for all time to come; if I transgress it and swear falsely, may the opposite of all this be my lot [3].

Although it is hard to prove, it is quite possible that the Greeks had built on what they learned from earlier civilisations, in particular the code of Hammurabi.

Many scientists see scientific research as separate from philosophical questions. Conversely, many philosophers see philosophy as separate from the results of science. Some philosophers, like Kant and pure rationalists like Descartes and Hegel, say that philosophy is better than science. They say that all philosophical problems can be solved without using science. They also say that science has to follow the framework that was discovered by philosophy alone. Richard Feynman, the famous physicist is reported to have said: 'Philosophy of science is about as useful to scientists as ornithology is to birds'. Logical positivists think that philosophy should be below science. They say that philosophy only helps by making better conceptual tools for scientists when they try to understand the world. The modern claim is that science and philosophy are overlapping disciplines that can benefit from interaction, but they are not identical. Often, the overlap is not important for specific research projects, but sometimes it is. And this is something that all scientists and science practitioners should know about.

This book has dual objectives. First, it aims to underscore the inherent philosophical dimension within medical science. Second, it seeks to emphasise that even practical and ethical medical issues can gain valuable insights from a philosophical perspective. By doing so, the book hopes to provide a much-needed resource for both the academic and non-academic readers. In the eleventh and twelfth centuries, the earliest European universities typically comprised four faculties: philosophy, medicine, law, and theology. Natural sciences were considered as branches of philosophy. Famous figures like Galileo and Newton did philosophical research, while philosophers like Descartes and Leibniz did important work in physics and math. In the Arab scientific-philosophical culture era, people like Ibn Sina and Ibn Rushd were excellent philosophers and doctors [3].

This is evident not only in the natural and medical sciences but also in many social sciences. During the European Middle Ages, people often sought authoritative answers from clergy members regarding questions about nature, humanity, and society. Sometimes, they even sought answers from clergy members regarding illnesses, as some illnesses were considered God's punishment.

Today, numerous economic, political, and administrative decisions, whether in public or private domains, rely on reports and recommendations from expert social scientists. Science has replaced religion as a major source of authority in the last two centuries. The combination of science, rationality, democracy, and industrialisation is often referred to as 'modernity'. Modernity contains a hitherto unseen stress on discussion and argumentation. Arguments are intended to convince, not just to persuade. This new way of thinking is what makes modernity so unique and exciting [3].

The main goal of studying bioethics is

1. Understand the basic principles of patient care and the medical profession.

2. Understanding common ethical issues such as informed consent, patient autonomy, end-of-life care, advanced care plan, and skills of effective communication.
3. Understand commonly encountered ethical issues in daily practice.
4. Competency for analysis and resolution of ethical problems.
5. Understanding diversity in cultural values and its impact on clinical decision-making.

References

1. Caplan AL. Does the philosophy of medicine exist? Theor Med. 1992;13:67–77.
2. Russell B. Ancient Philosophy, Part II. Socrates, Plato and Aristotle. Book One. Chapter XXII. Simon and Schuster; New York, NY: 1972. A History of Western Philosophy, 3. Oxtoby K. Is the Hippocratic oath still relevant to practising doctors today? BMJ. 2016;355:i6629. https://doi.org/10.1136/bmj.i6629.
3. Johansson I, Lynøe N. Medicine & philosophy. A twenty-first century introduction. Ontos Verlag. ISBN 978-3-938793-90-9. p. 1–5.

Chapter 4
Approach to Medical Ethics

> it is a great thing to die in your own bed, though it is better still to die in your boots. However great the kindness and efficiency, in every hospital death there will be some small, squalid detail, something perhaps too small to be told but leaving terribly painful memories behind, arising out of the haste, the overcrowding, the impersonality of a place where every day people are dying among strangers. (George Orwell)

Various disciplines and multidisciplinary approaches actively study medical ethics. In medical education, it primarily focuses on two key tasks. One involves teaching and learning the professional standards of competence and conducts expected by the medical profession—an endeavour shared with clinical teaching. The effectiveness of classroom instruction relies on reinforcement through practical examples. The second task centres on teaching and learning how to express and analyse the growing array of ethical dilemmas arising in medical practice, many of which lack clear or consensus-driven solutions [1].

Percival, a significant figure in the history of medicine, made notable contributions to the development of medical ethics. His work, particularly his book "Medical Ethics," aimed to establish ethical guidelines for healthcare professionals. Percival emphasised the importance of professionalism, moral conduct, and the physician's duty to prioritise the well-being of patients. His insights laid the groundwork for ethical considerations in medical practice. In 1803, he released his "Code of Institutes and Precepts adapted to the Professional Conduct of Physicians and Surgeons. This publication proved highly influential, particularly in the United States. Notably, the American Medical Association acknowledged the significant influence of Percival's work, with its 1847 "Code of Medical Ethics" largely deriving from his work [2].

A different answer to medical ethics came from John Gregory. Gregory not only delivered but also published a series of lectures titled "Lectures on the Duties and Qualifications of a Physician." These lectures were significant in shaping the perspectives and responsibilities expected of physicians during that era.

His emphasis on the duties and qualifications of a physician highlighted the importance of professionalism, ethics, and moral conduct. Gregory's teachings provided a foundational framework for understanding the broader role of physicians in

S. Abbas, *Medical Ethics*, https://doi.org/10.1007/978-981-96-9199-9_4

society, extending beyond medical expertise to include ethical considerations and interpersonal skills.

His teaching has become a valuable resource for medical practitioners and educators. His work contributed to the evolving discourse on medical ethics and professionalism, setting the stage for the development of ethical guidelines within the medical community. Gregory's legacy endures through the lasting impact of his teachings on the ethical dimensions of medical practice. While "no profession requires so comprehensive a mind as medicine," he said in the medical profession there was "no established authority to which we can refer in doubtful cases. Every physician must rest on his own judgment, which appeals for its rectitude to nature and experience alone." His vision for medical practice was farsighted and realised in the second half of the twentieth century, likely caused by the dramatic biomedical advances in the post–World War II period, advances in surgery such as in vitro fertilisation and organ transplant surgery [3]. By then there was more emphasis on what medicine can do and how to do it rather than what medicine can do.

Individuals who want to study medicine, require a comprehensive grasp of the clinical, scientific, and ethical considerations to autonomously make informed decisions and actively contribute to public discussions and decision-making processes. Consequently, doctors had to undergo a process of relearning effective communication, both with individual patients and in the realm of public opinion. They also needed to be willing to share not only their knowledge but also their uncertainties with patients and the public [1, 3].

The study of medical ethics is divided by Boyd into theoretical principles of moral theory, professionals and patients as moral agents and perspective-based approach focusing on the course of events [1].

Principles

In employing a principles-based approach, the central inquiry revolves around determining the moral correctness of a specific act or course of action. Its moral rightness is determined by its adherence to an established moral rule or the acknowledgment of an agreed moral principle. These rules or principles can be deontological, centred on duties and rights, or consequentialist, focusing on the consequences of the action. All principles-based approaches share the commonality that the action or course of action should align with an established moral rule or principle. Adhering to principles is better than acting without principles, but there is disagreement about which principles to follow. For example, people disagree about whether it is more important to follow the rules or do what you think is right. Both consequentialists and deontologists have debated this and defended their positions. Every principle is arguable and has to make adjustments or exceptions as dictated by events and the perspective of involved personnel. Each of the four pillars of ethics should be followed unless they contradict.

In essence, the issue with the four principles is that they do not offer a decision-making process for resolving conflicts or arriving at practical conclusions. In line with the principles of beneficence and non-maleficence, immediate treatment is deemed to bring more good than harm to the patient. However, if the patient refuses treatment, is evidently competent, and insists on exercising their autonomy, the treatment cannot be administered according to the principle of respect for autonomy [1–3].

Detractors of "principlism," as some philosophical critics refer to it, contend that these principles may function more as slogans, employed to endorse conclusions that have been reached without genuinely applying the principles in the decision-making process. The four principles can also be viewed as what is sometimes termed "regulative ideals" [4, 5].

People

Rooted in principles as ancient as those of Aristotle, this perspective redirects attention from the moral act to the moral agent. Commonly known as "virtue ethics," this approach is less preoccupied with determining the right action and more focused on cultivating the qualities that contribute to becoming the best kind of person [6].

Perspective

A perspectives-based approach initiates its examination by directing attention away from the specific action or the individual involved and instead centres its focus on the case at hand. In other words, rather than immediately delving into the ethical dimensions of the action or the character of the person involved, this approach begins by thoroughly examining the unique circumstances and details of the situation under consideration. By prioritising the case, it seeks to comprehend the nuanced factors and contextual elements that may influence ethical considerations, providing a comprehensive foundation for ethical analysis and decision-making. A perspectives-based approach acknowledges that a moral dilemma is not a predetermined entity, akin to a natural object. Instead, it is an interpretation of events viewed from a perspective influenced by history and tradition [1].

Similar to a clinical case, a moral dilemma is an interpretation assigned to events, viewed from a perspective influenced by history and tradition. This construction is not always a conscious one; rather, it often resides implicitly in language. For instance, when Orwell refers to a "small, squalid detail," a moral judgment or justification is already taking form:

"it is a great thing to die in your own bed, though it is better still to die in your boots. However great the kindness and efficiency, in every hospital death there will be some small, squalid detail, something perhaps too small to be told but leaving terribly painful memories behind, arising out of the haste, the overcrowding, the impersonality of a place where every day people are dying among strangers." . The demonstration that moral problems are not inherent or externally defined is evident in the phenomenon known as "moral blindness." This term refers to individuals who fail to recognise the existence of a moral dilemma, as seen in cases where, for instance, they may not perceive a moral issue in telling a lie if they believe they can escape consequences [1, 7]. Also cultures vary in their recognition of moral dilemmas and in their preferred methods of resolving moral issues. Each of us, influenced by our unique blend of tradition, education, and life experiences, holds distinct moral perspectives that may differ significantly from those of others.

Prejudicial Interpretation (Hermeneutics)

It often involves understanding the meaning and significance of complex or ambiguous phenomena. The goal of hermeneutics is to derive meaning and understanding from these phenomena by considering the context, historical background, and the interplay of different elements involved in the interpretation process. Hermeneutics has expanded its scope to encompass the interpretation of behaviour, speech, and institutions. Hans–Georg Gadamer, a prominent figure in hermeneutics, advocates for a favourable perspective on prejudice, prejudgment, or fore-understanding. According to him, these anticipations are essential, serving as the initial framework through which we begin to comprehend and engage with the information or perspectives presented to us. In Gadamer's view, without this preliminary projection of meaning, the process of understanding and connecting with a text or a person would be challenging to initiate. It is essential for deliberation, that when two people, each holding distinct viewpoints on a topic, engage in a conversation, they may ultimately develop a new, mutually shared perspective on the subject [8].

Approaching everyday ethical issues from a hermeneutic perspective is, at a minimum, integral to effective risk management. If executed successfully, it may also facilitate consensus among those involved regarding "a course of action likely to be responsive to more features of the situation, and thus more nuanced and efficacious." [9].

References

1. Boyd KM. Medical ethics: principles, persons, and perspectives: from controversy to conversation. J Med Ethics. 2005;31:481–6.
2. Leake CD, editor. Percival's medical ethics. Huntington, NY: Robert E Kreiger Publishing Company; 1975.
3. Gregory J. The duties and qualifications of a physician. In: Broadie A, editor. The Scottish enlightenment: an anthology. Edinburgh: Canongate; 1997. 760ff.
4. Gillon R, Lloyd A, editors. Principles of health care ethics. Chichester: Wiley; 1994.
5. Emmet D. The role of the unrealisable: a study in regulative ideals. Houndmills: Macmillan, St Martin's Press; 1994.

6. Hursthouse R. Virtue theory and abortion. In: Statman D, editor. Virtue ethics: a critical reader. Edinburgh: Edinburgh University Press; 1997. p. 230.
7. Orwell G. How the poor die. Collected essays. London: Mercury Books, Heinemann; 1961. 225
8. Gadamer H-G. Truth and method. London: Sheed and Ward; 1988. 235ff
9. Leder D. Toward a hermeneutic bioethics. In: DuBose ER, Hamel R, O'Connell LJ, editors. A matter of principles? Ferment in US bioethics. Valley Forge, PA: Trinity Press International; 1994. p. 240–59.

Chapter 5
Fundamental Principles of Medical Ethics

- Main principles of ethics
  - Beneficence
  - Non-maleficence
  - Autonomy: Autonomy is the basis for informed consent, sincerity, and patients' confidentiality
  - Justice
  - Avoiding conflict of interest
- A model of care that integrates
  - Ethics
  - Professionalism
  - Cognitive and technical expertise

The field of ethics rapidly evolved from its initial concern with professional conduct and codes to include research ethics, public health ethics, organisational ethics, and clinical ethics, reflecting its extensive contemporary scope. This transformation was driven by unfortunate abuses in research, medical interventions without informed consent, and experimentation during World War II. Simultaneously, significant advancements in medicine and technology, as well as societal changes, expanded bioethics to encompass research ethics, public health ethics, organisational ethics, and clinical ethics [1]. Ethics is the study of moral principles and decisions, and how to apply them. Normative ethics asks, "What moral standards should we use and why? What justifies our choices?" [2].

Certain moral principles for proper behaviour are universally shared by humanity, transcending cultural, regional, religious, and group distinctions. These principles form what is known as common morality. Examples include refraining from killing or causing harm to others, avoiding theft, not punishing the innocent, telling the truth, abiding by the law, caring for the young and dependent, aiding those in distress, and rescuing those in peril [2]. Particular morality is about norms that bind specific groups due to their culture, religion, profession, or other factors. For

S. Abbas, *Medical Ethics*, https://doi.org/10.1007/978-981-96-9199-9_5

example, physicians have a defined role to provide competent and reliable care to their patients. Physician organisations at the local, state, and national levels have established codified standards. However, it is important to recognise that adhering to these standards may not always align with broader moral principles, as these codes have at times seemed to prioritise the interests of the medical profession over offering a comprehensive moral perspective or addressing issues crucial to patients and society [3]. Bioethics has undergone rapid evolution, spurred by deplorable abuses in human subject research, medical interventions without informed consent, and experimentation during World War II. Simultaneously, advancements in medicine and medical technology, coupled with societal changes, have expanded bioethics beyond concerns about professional conduct and codes. It now encompasses a broad scope, including research ethics, public health ethics, organisational ethics, and clinical ethics.

The four principles of ethics in contemporary medical ethics are beneficence, non-maleficence, autonomy, and justice. The first two, "to help and do no harm," have their origins in the time of Hippocrates. In Percival's book on ethics in the early nineteenth century, the emphasis was on prioritising the patient's best interests. Autonomy and justice were not discussed at that time. However, over time, both autonomy and justice gained recognition and acceptance as essential ethical principles in the field of medicine. In today's society, patients have the right to make decisions about their bodies and their health care. Therefore, it is important for doctors to respect their patients' autonomy and the right to justice [2].

Beneficence

This principle underscores the moral obligation of physicians to act in the best interests of their patients. It encompasses several key moral rules:

1. Protect and Defend the Rights of Others: Physicians are ethically bound to safeguard the rights and well-being of their patients. This includes respecting their autonomy and ensuring that their decisions and choices are honoured.
2. Prevent Harm: Beneficence requires physicians to proactively avoid causing harm to their patients. This entails taking measures to reduce risks and protect the patient from adverse outcomes.
3. Remove Conditions that Cause Harm: Physicians should work to alleviate or eliminate conditions that are causing harm to the patient. This could involve diagnosing and treating diseases or addressing other health-related concerns.
4. Help Persons with Disabilities: Beneficence extends to assisting individuals with disabilities. Physicians should strive to enhance the quality of life and well-being of patients with disabilities, taking into account their specific needs and challenges.

5. Rescue Persons in Danger: In situations where patients are in imminent danger, physicians have an ethical duty to take action to rescue and provide care, if possible.

The principle of beneficence is characterised by its positive requirements. It does not merely advocate for the avoidance of harm but also emphasises actively promoting the welfare and well-being of patients. Physicians are encouraged to go beyond the duty of non-maleficence (not causing harm) and actively seek ways to benefit their patients.

Additionally, while physicians' beneficence is rooted in altruism and a commitment to patient well-being, it is worth considering that, in some cases, it can also be seen as a form of reciprocity. This can include a sense of repaying the societal investment in their education (often subsidised by governments), the privileges and ranks they hold within the medical profession, and the knowledge and skills they gain through patient interactions, which can contribute to medical learning and research.

In essence, the principle of beneficence underscores the proactive and positive role that physicians play in promoting the welfare of their patients while taking into account broader societal and ethical considerations [1–3].

Nonmaleficence: This principle is often summarised as the ethical obligation of a physician not to harm the patient. It is a foundational principle in medical ethics and encompasses several key moral rules:

1. Do Not Kill: Physicians are fundamentally obligated not to take actions that intentionally lead to the death of their patients. This includes refraining from actions that may result in euthanasia or assisted suicide, which are generally considered ethically and legally prohibited in many healthcare contexts.
2. Do Not Cause Pain or Suffering: Physicians must take all reasonable measures to prevent and alleviate pain and suffering in their patients. This involves the responsible management of pain and discomfort during medical procedures and treatments.
3. Do Not Incapacitate: Physicians should avoid actions that render patients incapacitated or unable to make autonomous decisions about their healthcare. Informed consent and respect for patient autonomy are vital components of this aspect of non-maleficence.
4. Do Not Cause Offence: Physicians should conduct themselves in a manner that does not cause unnecessary offence or harm to patients. This includes being respectful, considerate, and culturally sensitive in their interactions.
5. Do Not Deprive Others of the Goods of Life: This principle extends to ensuring that patients have access to the basic necessities and goods required for a dignified life, such as food, water, shelter, and medical care.

The practical application of the principle of non-maleficence involves a careful ethical analysis by the physician. They must weigh the potential benefits and burdens of all medical interventions and treatments. The goal is to choose the course of action that is most likely to promote the patient's well-being while minimising harm or suffering.

This principle is particularly relevant in challenging decisions related to end-of-life care. Physicians are often faced with dilemmas surrounding the withholding or withdrawing of life-sustaining treatments, decisions about medically administered nutrition and hydration, and the management of pain and other symptoms in terminally ill patients. In such cases, a physician's primary obligation is to relieve patient suffering. The doctrine of double effect acknowledges that in pursuing this goal, there may be foreseen but unintended harmful consequences. However, these harmful effects are ethically acceptable if they are a consequence of pursuing the primary aim of relieving suffering.

In summary, the principle of non-maleficence places a fundamental duty on physicians to avoid causing harm to their patients. It guides decisions about medical interventions and treatments, especially in complex end-of-life care scenarios, where the relief of suffering takes precedence while recognising the possibility of unintended, but ethically justifiable, negative outcomes [4, 5].

The court decision by Justice Benjamin Cardozo in 1914, often cited for its epigrammatic dictum, "Every human being of adult years and sound mind has a right to determine what shall be done with his own body," represents a significant legal and ethical principle in the realm of individual autonomy and bodily integrity.

This statement, often referred to as the principle of bodily autonomy, which places a strong emphasis on individual autonomy, recognising that competent adults have the right to make decisions about their own bodies. This includes choices related to medical treatments, procedures, and intervention, This principle is important in modern healthcare, where individuals have the right to make medical choices without coercion, and where individuals are given the opportunity to be informed about their options [6].

The philosophical underpinning for autonomy, as interpreted by philosophers Immanuel Kant and John Stuart Mill, serves as a foundational principle in ethics and has profound implications for personal freedom and decision-making.

Immanuel Kant (1724–1804)

Kant's ethical philosophy is often associated with the concept of autonomy. According to Kant, every individual possesses intrinsic and unconditional worth or dignity. This means that every person is valuable simply by virtue of being a rational human being, and this worth is not contingent on any external factors, such as social status or accomplishments.

Kant's ethical framework emphasises the importance of rationality and moral agency. He argues that individuals have the capacity for rational thought and moral reasoning, and this capacity gives them the power to make autonomous decisions and moral choices. Autonomy, in Kant's view, is the capacity to act in accordance with one's own rational will, free from external coercion or manipulation.

For Kant, autonomy is closely tied to the notion of moral duty and the categorical imperative, which is a universal moral law. According to the categorical imperative, individuals should act in a way that they can will their actions to become universal laws applicable to all rational beings. In other words, individuals should make moral choices based on principles that can be applied consistently to everyone [1].

John Stuart Mill (1806–1873)

John Stuart Mill's perspective on autonomy aligns with his utilitarian philosophy. Mill argues that individual autonomy is essential for maximising happiness and well-being in society. He contends that individuals are the best judges of their own interests and that they should have the freedom to pursue their own happiness as long as their actions do not harm others.

Mill's harm principle states that the only legitimate reason for interfering with an individual's autonomy is to prevent harm to others. This principle upholds the importance of personal liberty and the right to make choices based on one's own values and preferences.

In summary, the philosophical underpinning for autonomy, as interpreted by Kant and Mill, underscores the idea that all individuals possess intrinsic worth and should have the power to make rational and moral decisions. Autonomy is seen as a fundamental ethical principle that recognises the value of personal freedom, self-determination, and the ability to act in accordance with one's own rational will while respecting the boundaries of not causing harm to others. This concept of autonomy has profound implications for ethics, human rights, and the way we understand personal agency and moral responsibility in society [7].

Balancing Autonomy with Competing Principles

Autonomy is a fundamental ethical principle that recognises an individual's right to make decisions about their own life and healthcare. However, like all ethical principles, it is not absolute and must be weighed against competing moral principles and considerations. One of the key considerations in balancing autonomy is the potential for harm to others.

Limitations on Autonomy

1. Harm to Others: Autonomy does not grant individuals the right to take actions that directly harm others. For instance, if an autonomous action by a patient poses a significant risk of harm to another person or persons, it may be justifiable to limit that autonomy in order to prevent harm.
2. Lack of Capacity (Competence): Autonomy is predicated on an individual's capacity to make rational and informed decisions. It does not extend to individuals who lack this capacity due to various reasons. This includes:

   Infants and Children: Children are generally considered to lack full autonomy due to their developmental stage and limited capacity to understand complex medical decisions.

   Incompetence due to Mental or Physical Disorders: Individuals who, due to mental illness, cognitive impairment, or physical disability, are unable to understand the nature and consequences of their decisions may also be considered lacking capacity.

   Assessment of Capacity and Incompetence: Healthcare institutions and state governments have established policies and procedures to assess an individual's capacity to make healthcare decisions. This assessment is typically performed by healthcare professionals and takes into account the individual's ability to understand relevant information, appreciate the consequences of decisions, and communicate their preferences [8].

   Practical Consequences of Lack of Capacity: It is important to note that there may not always be a rigid distinction between a clinician's determination of a patient's lack of decision-making capacity based on physical or mental disorders and a legal determination of incompetence by a court of law. From a practical standpoint, both determinations can lead to similar consequences, such as the appointment of a legal guardian or surrogate decision-maker to act in the best interests of the individual.

While the principle of autonomy is a fundamental ethical tenet that upholds an individual's right to make choices about their healthcare, it is subject to limitations when it conflicts with the well-being of others or when individuals lack the capacity to make autonomous decisions. Balancing autonomy with competing moral principles and assessing capacity are complex ethical and practical challenges that healthcare professionals, institutions, and legal systems address to ensure the best interests and rights of individuals are upheld in healthcare decision-making [8].

Relational Autonomy

The principle of autonomy traditionally emphasises the individual's right to make decisions about their own life and healthcare, with a strong focus on personal values, preferences, and informed consent.

Detractors of the traditional view argue that autonomy is not solely an individualistic concept but is shaped and influenced by various social relationships and complex determinants such as gender, ethnicity, and culture. This perspective is often referred to as "relational autonomy."

Key Aspects of Relational Autonomy

Social Context

Relational autonomy recognises that an individual's autonomy is situated within a broader social context. Our values, choices, and preferences are often influenced by the relationships we have with family, community, and society.

Complex Determinants

This view acknowledges that factors like gender, ethnicity, and culture can play a significant role in shaping an individual's autonomy. Different cultural backgrounds and societal norms can lead to diverse perspectives on healthcare decision-making.

Interdependence

Relational autonomy highlights the interdependence of individuals within their social networks. It considers how the autonomy of one person may be intertwined with the autonomy and well-being of others, especially in familial and communal contexts.

Cultural Diversity and Autonomy

In countries like the United States, which have culturally diverse populations, the concept of autonomy is not uniform across all groups. Some minority populations may hold views and values that differ from the majority population, particularly in healthcare decision-making.

For example, in some cultures, decision-making about healthcare is seen as a collective or family-centred process, where the preferences of the family unit carry significant weight. This contrasts with the more individualistic approach to autonomy prevalent in Western bioethics.

Implications

Relational autonomy challenges the one-size-fits-all approach to autonomy in healthcare ethics. It recognises the need for cultural competence and sensitivity in healthcare delivery.

It also raises questions about how healthcare professionals should navigate situations where the individual's autonomy may be influenced by family dynamics or cultural norms that prioritise communal decision-making.

Balancing Individual and Relational Autonomy

In practice, healthcare providers often need to navigate the complex terrain of individual and relational autonomy. This may involve respecting the individual's autonomy while acknowledging and involving family members or community representatives in the decision-making process when appropriate.

Ethical discussions often revolve around finding a balance between respecting individual choices and recognising the influence of relational and cultural factors.

In summary, detractors of the principle of autonomy advocate for a broader concept of relational autonomy that acknowledges the influence of social relationships, culture, and complex determinants on individual decision-making. This perspective highlights the need for healthcare professionals to be culturally sensitive and attuned to the diverse ways in which autonomy is understood and practiced within different communities and populations [1, 9, 10].

Resistance to the principle of patient autonomy remains problematic, especially in non-western cultures, also in the west there is a need for a critical examination of paternalistic medical practices in light of changing cultural, technological, and societal trends.

Resistance to Patient Autonomy in Non-western Cultures

The principle of patient autonomy, which underscore an individual's right to make decisions about their own healthcare, has been a fundamental tenet of Western bioethics. However, this principle may face resistance in non-western cultures with ancient civilisations and deeply rooted beliefs and traditions.

In these cultures, physicians may practice paternalism, where they make decisions in what they believe to be the best interest of the patient, often without seeking explicit patient consent. Paternalism is rooted in the principle of beneficence, the obligation to act in the patient's best interest.

This resistance to patient autonomy can be attributed to cultural norms and the belief that healthcare decisions should be made collectively or guided by family or community elders [1, 3].

Changing Nature of Culture

Culture is not static but evolves over time. It is influenced by various factors, including technological advancements, economic progress, changes in education and socioeconomic status, globalisation, and evolving societal values.

As societies undergo these transformations, traditional patterns and roles in physician–patient relationships may no longer hold true. There is a shift towards emphasising the patient as an individual with unique values and preferences, rather than just as a member of a group or family.

Need for Critical Examination

Given the evolving cultural landscape and changing dynamics in healthcare, a critical examination of paternalistic medical practices is necessary.

This examination should include research efforts, such as well-structured surveys, to understand demographics, patient preferences regarding informed consent, truth-telling, and the patient's role in decision-making.

Research can provide valuable insights into how cultural attitudes towards healthcare decision-making are evolving and how healthcare systems can adapt to meet the changing needs and expectations of patients.

It is critical to understand cultural diversity in healthcare and the need for healthcare practices to evolve in response to changing cultural, technological, and societal trends. This calls for research as a means to better understand and navigate the complex interplay among patient autonomy, cultural beliefs, and evolving healthcare systems [1, 4].

Respecting the principle of autonomy in healthcare obliges physicians to engage in certain practices, such as disclosing medical information, ensuring informed consent, truth-telling, and maintaining confidentiality:

Disclosure of Medical Information

Respecting patient autonomy involves providing patients with relevant and comprehensible medical information about their condition, diagnosis, treatment options, risks, benefits, and potential outcomes.

This disclosure allows patients to make informed decisions about their healthcare based on a clear understanding of the situation and available choices.

Physicians have a duty to ensure that the information provided is accurate, up-to-date, and tailored to the patient's level of understanding. Effective communication is essential to meet this obligation.

Informed Consent

Informed consent is a fundamental component of respecting patient autonomy. It means that patients have the right to make voluntary and informed decisions about their medical treatment.

Physicians must obtain the patient's explicit consent before initiating any treatment or medical procedure. This process involves explaining the proposed treatment, potential risks and benefits, alternatives, and allowing the patient to ask questions.

Informed consent ensures that patients are actively involved in their healthcare decisions and have the autonomy to accept or refuse medical interventions.

Truth-Telling

Respecting patient autonomy includes a commitment to truth-telling. Physicians have an ethical obligation to provide patients with accurate and honest information about their medical condition, prognosis, and treatment options.

This truth-telling fosters trust between patients and healthcare providers, empowers patients to make informed choices, and upholds the principle of autonomy. It also allows patients to plan for their future based on realistic expectations.

Confidentiality

Respecting patient autonomy extends to maintaining patient confidentiality. Physicians must safeguard the privacy of medical information and protect sensitive patient data.

Patients must feel confident that their personal health information will not be disclosed without their consent, except when required by law or for the purpose of providing appropriate care.

Upholding confidentiality helps build trust in the physician–patient relationship, which is essential for open and honest communication.

Respecting the principle of autonomy in healthcare involves a range of ethical obligations on the part of physicians. These obligations include providing clear and accurate medical information, obtaining informed consent, being truthful with patients, and maintaining the confidentiality of patient records. By adhering to these practices, healthcare professionals empower patients to make autonomous decisions about their health and well-being, ensuring that their values, preferences, and choices are respected in the healthcare process [1, 4, 9].

The requirements of informed consent for medical or surgical procedures and research, each of which is designed to ensure that the patient or research subject is fully informed and able to make autonomous decisions:

Competence to Understand and Decide

The first requirement of informed consent is that the individual must be competent. Competence means that the person has the mental capacity to understand the relevant information and make decisions about their healthcare or participation in research.

Healthcare providers or researchers typically assess a person's competence based on their ability to comprehend information, weigh the risks and benefits, and communicate their decisions. If a person is deemed incompetent due to cognitive impairment or other factors, a legal guardian or surrogate decision-maker may be involved in the consent process. Since competence is the initial requirement for informed consent, it is essential to understand how to identify incompetence. Accepted standards, which can be used individually or in combination, for assessing incompetence typically revolve around the patient's incapacity to express a preference or decision, inability to comprehend their circumstances and the potential outcomes, and incapacity to logically process significant life choices.

Full Disclosure

Full disclosure means providing the patient or research subject with all relevant information about the medical or research procedure. This includes details about the nature of the procedure, its purpose, potential risks and benefits, available alternatives, and the expected outcome.

The information should be presented in a clear and understandable manner, free from jargon, and tailored to the individual's level of comprehension. It is essential that no important information is withheld.

Comprehension of Disclosure

It is not sufficient to merely provide information; the individual must also comprehend the disclosed information. Healthcare providers or researchers should assess whether the patient or subject understands the information presented to them.

This assessment may involve asking the person to explain the procedure, its risks, and its potential consequences in their own words. If there is any doubt about comprehension, additional explanations or educational materials may be provided.

Voluntary Decision-Making

Informed consent requires that the decision to proceed with a medical procedure or participate in research is made voluntarily, free from coercion, pressure, or undue influence. The individual must be able to make the decision without feeling forced or manipulated.

Physicians, researchers, or healthcare providers should respect the individual's autonomy and allow them sufficient time to consider their options and ask questions. Decisions should not be rushed or coerced.

Consent to the Proposed Action

Finally, informed consent involves obtaining explicit consent from the patient or research subject to proceed with the proposed action. This means the individual agrees, based on their understanding of the information provided, to undergo the medical procedure or participate in the research study.

Consent can be given either in writing (signed informed consent forms) or verbally, depending on local regulations and institutional policies.

Informed consent is a critical ethical and legal requirement in medical practice and research. It ensures that individuals are fully informed about their healthcare or research participation, have the capacity to make decisions, voluntarily consent to the proposed action, and are protected from coercion or manipulation. These requirements are designed to uphold the principle of autonomy and respect the individual's right to make informed choices about their own health and involvement in research [11, 12].

Let's elaborate on the complex decision-making processes involved in cases where a previously autonomous patient becomes incompetent and requires a surrogate decision-maker:

Respecting Previously Expressed Preferences

When a patient who was previously autonomous and capable of making their own decisions becomes incompetent, their previously expressed preferences or autonomous judgments should be respected. These preferences are seen as a reflection of the patient's prior autonomous choices and values.

Respecting these preferences acknowledges the patient's autonomy even in their current state of incompetence. It ensures that the patient's wishes, as they were when competent, guide their medical care.

Surrogate Decision-Maker for Incompetent Patients

In situations where a patient is currently incompetent, whether due to a temporary condition or cognitive decline, a surrogate decision-maker is required to make healthcare decisions on their behalf.

There are two commonly used standards for surrogate decision-making:

Substituted Judgment Standard: This standard involves the surrogate making decisions based on what the patient would have chosen in the current circumstances if they were still competent. It prioritises the patient's previously expressed preferences over the surrogate's own preferences.

Best Interests Standard: This standard requires the surrogate to make decisions that are in the patient's best interests, considering factors such as medical evidence, potential benefits, and risks. It aims to promote the patient's overall well-being.

1. The Concept of "Substituted Interests".

In cases where the surrogate is uncertain about the patient's preferences or when the patient's preferences may not align with current medical knowledge or advances, the concept of "substituted interests" can be applied.

"Substituted interests" involve determining the patient's authentic values and interests, even if their specific preferences are unclear. This approach seeks to make decisions that align with the patient's core values and what would have mattered most to them.

It provides a practical option for surrogates when the patient's prior preferences are not well-documented or when the medical context has evolved since those preferences were expressed.

The decision-making process for previously autonomous but presently incompetent patients involves a careful balance of respecting their prior preferences, appointing a surrogate decision-maker, and applying appropriate standards (substituted judgment or best interests) based on the circumstances. The concept of "substituted interests" offers an additional approach when patient preferences are unclear or outdated, aiming to make decisions that align with the patient's fundamental values and interests. These principles aim to uphold the patient's autonomy and well-being even in situations of incapacity [13, 14].

The truth-telling in the physician–patient relationship and the role of patient autonomy in this context: The patient's right to information about their health is an important part of the doctor–patient relationship, and the doctor is responsible for providing the patient with accurate information. The doctor should be honest and transparent with the patient about their health and any treatment options, and the patient should be able to make decisions about their own health care. The patient's right to information about their health is an important part of the doctor–patient relationship, and the doctor is responsible for providing the patient with accurate information. The doctor should be honest and transparent with the patient about their health and any treatment options, and the patient should be able to make decisions about their own health care.

Truth-Telling and Trust

Truth-telling is a fundamental and indispensable element in the physician-patient relationship. The foundation of this relationship is built on trust, and trust is closely tied to the honesty and transparency of the healthcare provider.

Patients rely on physicians not only for medical expertise but also for accurate information about their health. When physicians are truthful and provide clear and honest information, patients are more likely to trust their healthcare recommendations and decisions.

Patient Autonomy and Disclosure

Patient autonomy emphasises the individual's right to make decisions about their own healthcare. This includes the right to know and understand their diagnosis, prognosis, treatment options, risks, and potential outcomes. This process is known as disclosure.

An autonomous patient has the right to receive this information and make informed choices based on it. However, autonomy also means having the option to decline or forgo this disclosure if the patient wishes not to receive specific details about their condition.

Respecting Patient Preferences

Respecting patient autonomy involves understanding and adhering to the patient's preferences regarding disclosure. Some patients may want to receive detailed information about their condition, while others may prefer not to know the specifics.

It is the physician's responsibility to ascertain the patient's preference regarding disclosure. This may involve having a conversation with the patient, asking open-ended questions, and creating a safe and non-judgmental space for the patient to express their wishes.

Balancing Disclosure and Autonomy

The challenge for healthcare providers is to strike a balance between providing necessary medical information and respecting the patient's autonomy. This means tailoring the level of disclosure to meet the patient's individual needs and preferences.

Some patients may want full and detailed information to actively participate in their healthcare decisions, while others may prefer a more limited disclosure to reduce anxiety or stress.

Truth-telling is a cornerstone of the physician–patient relationship, underpinned by trust. Patient autonomy grants individuals the right to receive medical information, but it also includes the option to decline this disclosure. Physicians must respect these preferences and ascertain whether a patient wants to know the specifics of their diagnosis and prognosis or prefers a more limited disclosure. This delicate balance ensures that healthcare decisions align with the patient's values and autonomy while maintaining trust and open communication in the physician-patient relationship [1, 2, 4].

The gradual shift from a culture of significant resistance to full disclosure of medical diagnoses to the current norm of transparency.

Historical Perspective

In the past, the practice of fully disclosing a medical diagnosis, no matter how serious the disease, was not the norm in the United States. Physicians often hesitate to provide patients with complete information about their health conditions.

Resistance to Full Disclosure

Significant resistance to full disclosure was highly prevalent among physicians. They were often hesitant to disclose a diagnosis, possibly due to concerns about how patients would emotionally handle the news, fear of causing distress, or a belief that withholding information was in the patient's best interest.

Shift in Physician Attitudes

A marked shift has occurred in the attitudes of physicians regarding full disclosure. This shift is evident in survey data:

In 1961, a survey indicated that 88% of physicians preferred to avoid disclosing a diagnosis to their patients.

By 1979, however, a significant transformation had taken place, with 98% of surveyed physicians favouring the disclosure of diagnoses.

Factors Contributing to the Shift

Several factors have contributed to this significant shift in physician attitudes:

Educational Progress: Medical education has evolved to emphasise the importance of open communication and patient-centred care. Physicians are now trained to recognise the value of disclosing diagnoses and engaging in shared decision-making with patients.

Socioeconomic Progress: Societal values and expectations have changed over time, with an increased emphasis on patient autonomy, empowerment, and the right to know about one's health.

Accountability: Physicians today are more accountable to society and regulatory bodies. Ethical standards and guidelines promote transparency and informed consent, reinforcing the importance of disclosure.

Awareness of Transgressions: The medical profession has become more aware of past clinical and research transgressions, which have highlighted the ethical imperative of full disclosure.

The shift from resistance to full disclosure to the current norm of openness in the United States can be attributed to a combination of educational advancements, societal changes, increased accountability, and a growing awareness of the ethical and moral obligations of healthcare providers. Physicians now recognise that fully disclosing diagnoses is not only in line with ethical principles but also essential for respecting patient autonomy and building trust in the physician-patient relationship. This transformation reflects a broader commitment to patient-centred care and ethical medical practice [15].

Surveys conducted in the United States consistently reveal that patients facing serious illnesses, such as cancer and other life-threatening diseases, express a strong desire to be fully informed about their medical conditions, including their diagnoses and prognoses. This preference reflects the profound significance of healthcare information in the lives of patients and their families.

Patient-Centred Care

Patient-centred care places the patient's needs, preferences, and values at the forefront of healthcare decision-making. It recognises that patients have the right to be active participants in their healthcare journeys.

Patients often view a clear understanding of their diagnosis and prognosis as a fundamental aspect of this patient-centred approach. They want to make informed decisions about their treatment, care options, and future plans.

The Ethical Imperative

Providing complete information about a diagnosis and prognosis, done with tact and sensitivity, should be the standard practice in healthcare. It aligns with fundamental ethical principles such as respect for autonomy and beneficence.

Honesty and transparency in medical communication not only uphold ethical standards but also contribute to building trust between healthcare providers and patients. Trust is essential for effective healthcare delivery.

The Consequences of Truth-Telling

Failing to disclose the truth about a cancer diagnosis can have profound and far-reaching consequences for patients and their families.

Completion of Important Life-Tasks: Patients who are aware of their diagnosis have the opportunity to engage in crucial life-tasks. They can provide guidance to loved ones, express their feelings, and say their goodbyes. Financial matters, including the division of assets, can be addressed, ensuring a smoother transition for family members. Reconciliation with estranged family and friends becomes possible.

Spiritual and Emotional Preparedness: Disclosure allows patients to attain spiritual and emotional order through reflection, prayer, rituals, and religious sacraments. This spiritual preparedness can provide comfort and solace during a challenging time.

The Human Aspect of Healthcare

Beyond medical treatments and procedures, healthcare encompasses the deeply human aspects of life, including relationships, emotions, and personal beliefs. Recognising and respecting these aspects is an integral part of holistic patient care.

The desire of patients to be fully informed about their diagnoses and prognoses should be honoured as a cornerstone of patient-centred care. Physicians and healthcare providers have a moral and ethical obligation to provide this information sensitively and honestly. This approach not only respects patient autonomy but also allows patients to engage in critical life-tasks, achieve emotional and spiritual preparedness, and maintain trust in their healthcare providers. It recognises that healthcare is not just about treating diseases but also about supporting individuals and their families through some of life's most challenging moments [16, 17].

The practice of physicians in non-western societies disclosing medical information to the patient's family rather than directly to the patient, along with the underlying reasons and the nuances of patient autonomy:

Physician-Family Disclosure Pattern

In many non-Western societies, a recurring practice is for physicians to communicate medical information, especially bad news, primarily to the patient's family rather than directly to the patient. This pattern contrasts with the Western practice of direct patient-physician communication.

Reasons for Physician Resistance to Direct Patient Disclosure

Several factors contribute to physicians' hesitancy to convey distressing information directly to patients:

Concern for Emotional Impact: Physicians may worry that delivering bad news directly to the patient could provoke anxiety, despair, or a loss of hope. They might want to shield the patient from immediate emotional distress.

Uncertainty about Outcomes: In some cases, physicians might not have complete certainty about the medical outcome or prognosis. They may fear that providing incomplete or uncertain information could lead to confusion or misunderstanding.

Perceived Patient Capability: There's a belief that the patient may not possess the cognitive or emotional capacity to comprehend the information or may prefer not to know the full details of their condition.

Patient Autonomy and Nuanced Decision-Making

The practice of involving the patient's family in medical discussions does not necessarily have to be a binary choice that excludes patient autonomy.

Autonomous Choice as a Patient Right: The principle of autonomy underscores that patients have the right to make decisions about their own healthcare, including the choice of who should be involved in their medical discussions.

Empowering Patients: In exercising their autonomy, patients may choose to authorise one or more family members to participate in medical discussions and decision-making on their behalf. This approach aligns with cultural norms and individual preferences while respecting the patient's right to be informed.

Cultural Sensitivity and Inclusivity

Healthcare providers in non-western societies can strike a balance by being culturally sensitive and inclusive. They can offer patients the option of involving family members in discussions while ensuring that the patient's voice and preferences are heard and respected.

Shared decision-making models that incorporate both patient and family input can foster a collaborative approach to healthcare.

The practice of physicians in non-western societies to disclose medical information to the patient's family rather than the patient directly reflects cultural norms and concerns about emotional impact and uncertainty. However, it is essential to recognise that patient autonomy remains a fundamental principle, and patients have the right to choose how they wish to be informed and who should be involved in their medical discussions. Healthcare providers can adopt nuanced approaches that honour cultural values while upholding patients' autonomy and ensuring that their voices are heard in matters of their own healthcare [18].

Patient Confidentiality

Patient confidentiality is a fundamental ethical and legal principle in healthcare. It obligates physicians to safeguard any confidential information disclosed by a patient, including medical history, diagnoses, and treatment plans.

The Exception of Necessary Sharing for Patient Care

An important exception to patient confidentiality arises when sharing medical information is necessary for the patient's care. This typically involves the primary physician sharing pertinent medical details with consultants, specialists, and healthcare teams involved in the patient's treatment.

This exception is based on implied patient authorisation, as it serves the patient's best interests by ensuring coordinated and comprehensive healthcare.

Challenges to Confidentiality in Modern Healthcare

In modern healthcare settings, especially in large hospitals with multiple departments and electronic medical records, maintaining strict patient confidentiality can be challenging.

The use of electronic health records necessitates a high level of security to protect patient data from unauthorised access or breaches.

Physician Responsibility for Confidentiality

Individual physicians play a crucial role in upholding patient confidentiality. It is their ethical duty to refrain from discussing specific patient cases with family members, friends, or in social gatherings.

The advent of social media has introduced new challenges to confidentiality. Physicians must exercise caution and avoid sharing patient-specific information on social platforms, which could violate privacy laws and ethical standards.

Noteworthy Exceptions to Confidentiality

While patient confidentiality is generally inviolable, there are specific situations where healthcare providers may breach confidentiality due to legal or ethical considerations:

Legally Required Reporting: Healthcare providers may be legally obligated to report certain conditions or events, such as gunshot wounds or certain infectious diseases, to public health authorities.

Protection of Others: In exceptional circumstances where maintaining confidentiality may cause significant harm to another individual or the public, there may be a duty to disclose information. For example, in cases of epidemics or partner notification in HIV disease, the greater public health interest may take precedence.

Balancing Privacy and Public Interest

The ethical challenge lies in balancing the patient's right to privacy and the broader public interest or the welfare of potential at-risk individuals.

These exceptions are typically guided by legal requirements and ethical principles that emphasise the protection of public health and safety.

Patient confidentiality remains a paramount principle in healthcare, ensuring trust and privacy between patients and healthcare providers. While there are exceptions that permit the sharing of medical information for patient care or in specific legally required situations, healthcare professionals must exercise diligence in safeguarding patient confidentiality, especially in an era of electronic medical records and social media. Striking the right balance between privacy and public interest is an ongoing ethical challenge in modern healthcare practice [19].

Justice in Clinical Ethics

Justice in clinical ethics pertains to the fair, equitable, and appropriate treatment of individuals within the healthcare system. It is an essential ethical principle that guides how healthcare resources, benefits, and burdens are allocated among patients and within the healthcare system.

Distributive Justice

Distributive justice is a specific category of justice that is highly relevant in clinical ethics. It concerns the principles and mechanisms governing the fair distribution of healthcare resources, including but not limited to:

Access to medical care and treatments.
Allocation of healthcare funding and resources.
Equitable distribution of medical technologies and interventions.
Fairness in healthcare policy development.
Principles of Distributive Justice.

Distributive justice operates on principles that aim to ensure fair and impartial resource allocation:

Equity: Equity suggests that healthcare resources should be distributed based on individual needs, without discrimination or bias. It emphasises providing care to those who need it most urgently or have the greatest health disparities.

Equality: Equality advocates for the equal distribution of healthcare resources among all individuals, regardless of their health status or other factors. It promotes equal access to essential healthcare services.

Need: The principle of need emphasises directing resources to those with the most significant health needs. It prioritises individuals whose health conditions require immediate attention or intensive care.

Utility: Utility-based allocation considers maximising the overall benefit to society. It involves allocating resources to interventions that offer the greatest health outcomes or value for the healthcare system.

Justified Norms and Social Cooperation

Distributive justice relies on justified norms, which are ethical guidelines and regulations that determine how healthcare resources are allocated. These norms are developed through a consensus of stakeholders, including healthcare professionals, policymakers, and the broader community.

The aim of distributive justice is to structure the terms of social cooperation in healthcare. It seeks to create a system where resources are allocated in a manner that promotes the common good, minimises disparities, and ensures that individuals receive appropriate care based on ethical principles.

Balancing Act

Achieving distributive justice in healthcare can be a complex and challenging endeavour. It often involves balancing competing interests, including individual rights, societal well-being, and resource constraints.

Ethical dilemmas may arise when resources are scarce, and decisions must be made regarding the allocation of treatments, organ transplants, or access to experimental therapies.

Justice in clinical ethics, particularly distributive justice, emphasises the fair, equitable, and appropriate distribution of healthcare resources. This principle seeks to ensure that healthcare benefits and burdens are allocated according to ethical principles and justified norms, ultimately promoting the common good and societal cooperation within the healthcare system. Balancing the diverse interests and needs of individuals and society is an ongoing ethical challenge in healthcare resource allocation [20].

Applying Principles of Distributive Justice

Equal Share: Distributing healthcare resources equally means that each person receives the same allocation of resources, regardless of their individual circumstances. This principle promotes fairness in access but may not account for variations in healthcare needs.

According to Need: Allocating resources according to need prioritises individuals with the greatest health requirements. It ensures that those in critical conditions or with severe health disparities receive more resources. However, defining "need" can be challenging, and it may lead to resource allocation disputes.

According to Effort: This principle allocates resources based on an individual's effort or lifestyle choices that impact health. It rewards individuals who actively maintain their health but could be seen as punitive to those with health challenges beyond their control.

According to Contribution: Allocating resources according to an individual's contribution to society or the healthcare system rewards those who have made significant contributions. However, it might overlook the needs of individuals who cannot contribute due to circumstances.

According to Merit: Merit-based distribution rewards individuals based on their personal achievements or attributes. While it encourages excellence, it might not address health disparities or prioritise those with limited opportunities.

According to Free-Market Exchanges: In a free-market healthcare system, resources are allocated based on individuals' ability to pay and the market demand for services. This principle can lead to unequal access based on financial status.

Challenges in Distributing Medical Resources

Balancing Principles: The challenge in achieving distributive justice lies in finding a balanced approach that considers multiple principles simultaneously. Healthcare allocation often requires a combination of these principles to address the diverse needs of individuals and promote fairness.

Resource Scarcity: When resources are limited, difficult decisions must be made about who receives care. These decisions may involve trade-offs between principles, such as prioritising need over equality or merit over effort.

Defining Criteria: Defining criteria for need, effort, contribution, or merit can be subjective and open to interpretation. Different stakeholders may have varying views on what constitutes these criteria, leading to ethical dilemmas.

Complex Decision-Making: Allocating healthcare resources often involves complex decision-making processes that consider medical urgency, available resources, patient preferences, and societal values. Ethical committees and guidelines are sometimes used to assist in these decisions.

Resource Allocation Policies: Healthcare institutions and governments develop resource allocation policies that aim to balance these principles. These policies may evolve over time as societal values and healthcare priorities change.

Ethical Considerations

Ethical debates and discussions are essential in healthcare resource allocation. Transparency, inclusivity, and public input in decision-making processes can help ensure that resource allocation aligns with societal values and ethics.

Achieving distributive justice in healthcare resource allocation involves considering various principles, often in combination, to balance fairness and effectiveness. The complexity lies in defining criteria, making challenging decisions in resource-limited situations, and adapting allocation policies to evolving ethical standards and societal needs. Ethical dialogue and transparent decision-making processes are crucial in addressing these challenges [1, 4, 20].

There are challenges and ethical considerations associated with the principle of distributive justice in various aspects of healthcare:

Allotment of Scarce Resources: Allocating scarce medical resources, such as life-saving equipment, diagnostic tests, medications, and organ transplants, raises ethical dilemmas. The principle of distributive justice necessitates fair and equitable distribution. However, in reality, resources are often limited, and decisions must be made about who will receive them. Ethical considerations include determining allocation criteria (e.g., medical need, prognosis, potential benefit), ensuring transparency in decision-making, and minimising biases.

Care of Uninsured Patients: Providing care to uninsured or underinsured patients is another aspect of distributive justice. Physicians and healthcare institutions face ethical questions about whether they should prioritise patients based on their ability to pay. Ethical considerations involve providing necessary care to all patients, regardless of their financial status, and advocating for policies that address healthcare disparities.

Allotment of Time for Outpatient Visits: In outpatient settings, physicians must manage their time efficiently to accommodate all patients. Ethical dilemmas arise when deciding how to allot time for visits. Should every patient receive equal time, or should time allocation be based on medical need, complexity of the case, or social and economic status? Ethical considerations include ensuring that patients with complex or critical health issues receive the time and attention they require, while also respecting the needs of all patients.

Conflicts of Interest: The principle of fairness takes on paramount importance in situations involving conflicts of interest. Physicians must prioritise the best interests of their patients above personal gain. For example, it is ethically unacceptable for a physician to choose a treatment option solely because it brings them financial benefit, especially when there are equally effective but less expensive alternatives. This underscores the importance of maintaining the patient's trust and well-being as the primary ethical duty.

Transparency and Accountability: To uphold the principle of distributive justice, healthcare institutions and physicians should establish transparent allocation criteria and decision-making processes. Transparency ensures that patients and the public can understand how resource allocation decisions are made. Accountability mechanisms can help prevent biases, conflicts of interest, and unfair practices.

Advocacy for Ethical Healthcare Policies: Physicians also have a role in advocating for healthcare policies and reforms that promote distributive justice. This may involve advocating for increased access to care, improved insurance coverage, and the equitable distribution of healthcare resources at a systemic level.

The principle of distributive justice in healthcare encompasses various ethical challenges, including resource allocation, care of underserved populations, time management in clinical practice, conflicts of interest, and the need for transparency and accountability. Physicians and healthcare institutions must navigate these challenges while upholding their ethical obligation to prioritise patient well-being and fairness in healthcare delivery [21].

References

1. Varkey B. Principles of clinical ethics and their application to practice. Med Princ Pract. 2021;30(1):17–28.
2. Beauchamp TL, Childress JF. Principles of bioethics. 7th ed. Oxford University Press; 2013.
3. Berkman ND, Wynia MK, Churchill LR. Gaps, conflicts, and consensus in the ethics statements of professional associations, medical groups, and health plans. J Med Ethics. 2004;30(4):395–401.

4. Beauchamp TL, Childress JF. Principles of biomedical ethics. New York, NY: Oxford University Press; 2009. p. 162–4.
5. Mularski RA, Puntillo K, Varkey B, Erstad BL, Grap MJ, Gilbert HC, et al. Pain management within the palliative and end-of-life care experience in the ICU. Chest. 2009;135(5):1360–9.
6. Cardozo B. Basic right to consent to medical care- Schlendorff vs the Society of the New York Hospital, 211 NY 125 105 NE 92 1914 LEXUS 1028; 1914.
7. Guyer P. Kant on the theory and practice of autonomy. Soc Philos Policy. 2003;20(2):70–98.
8. Grisso T, Appelbaum PS. Assessing competence to consent to treatment: a guide to physicians and other health professionals. New York: Oxford University Press; 1998. p. 11.
9. Blackhall LJ, Murphy ST, Frank G, Michel V, Azen S. Ethnicity and attitudes toward patient autonomy. JAMA. 1995;274(10):820–5.
10. Mackenzie CM, Stoljar N. Relational autonomy: feminist perspectives on autonomy, agency, and the social self. New York: Oxford University Press; 2000.
11. Angell M. Ethical imperialism? Ethics in international collaborative clinical research. N Engl J Med. 1988;319(16):1081–3.
12. Appelbaum PS, Grisso T. Assessing patients' capacities to consent to treatment. N Engl J Med. 1988;319(25):1635–8.
13. Sulmasy DP, Snyder L. Substituted interests and best judgments: an integrated model of surrogate decision making. JAMA. 2010;304(17):1946–7.
14. Davis JK. The concept of precedent autonomy. Bioethics. 2002;16(2):114–33.
15. Novack DH, Plumer R, Smith RL, Ochitill H, Morrow GR, Bennett JM. Changes in physicians' attitudes toward telling the cancer patient. JAMA. 1979;241(9):897–900.
16. Rayson D. A piece of my mind. Lisa's stories. JAMA. 1999;282(17):1605–6.
17. Fallowfield LJ, Jenkins VA, Beveridge HA. Truth may hurt but deceit hurts more: communication in palliative care. Palliat Med. 2002;16(4):297–303.
18. Surbone A. Truth telling to the patient. JAMA. 1992;268(13):1661–2.
19. Weiss BD. Confidentiality expectations of patients, physicians, and medical students. JAMA. 1982;247(19):2695–7.
20. Fleishacker S. A short history of distributive justice. Cambridge, MA: Harvard University Press; 2005.
21. ABIM Foundation, American Board of Internal MedicineACP-ASIM Foundation, American College of Physicians-American Society of Internal MedicineEuropean Federation of Internal Medicine. Medical professionalism in the new millennium: a physician charter. Ann Intern Med. 2002;136(3):243–6.

Chapter 6
Conflicts Between Principles

The application of the four principles of ethics in medical decision can be complex and results in conflicts that may arise when these principles intersect. Let us break it down step by step:

Four Principles of Ethics: In the field of medical ethics, four fundamental principles are often used as a framework for ethical decision-making. These principles are:

Beneficence: The principle of doing good and promoting the well-being of the patient.

Non-maleficence: The principle of not causing harm to the patient.

Autonomy: Respecting the patient's right to make decisions about their own medical treatment, even if those decisions are contrary to medical advice.

Justice: Ensuring fairness and equality in the distribution of healthcare resources and access to medical care.

Prima Facie Obligations: Each of these four principles is considered a prima facie obligation, meaning that they must be fulfilled unless there is a conflict with another principle in a specific instance. Prima facie obligations are duties that are initially binding but can be overridden by more pressing moral considerations.

Conflict Resolution: When a conflict arises between these principles in a specific medical scenario, it becomes the physician's responsibility to determine the actual obligation to the patient. This determination involves assessing the relative importance or weight of the competing prima facie obligations based on both the content of the principles and the context of the situation.

Example of an Easy Resolution: Example where the principle of beneficence (doing what is best for the patient) overrides the principle of non-maleficence (avoiding harm). In this case, a patient in shock needs urgent fluid resuscitation, even though the placement of an intravenous catheter causes pain and swelling. The immediate priority is saving the patient's life, so the principle of beneficence takes precedence.

Complex Conflicts: Many conflicts in medical ethics are much more complex and difficult to resolve. It offers two specific scenarios:

S. Abbas, *Medical Ethics*, https://doi.org/10.1007/978-981-96-9199-9_6

Competent Patient's Refusal: When a competent patient refuses a potentially life-saving intervention, such as mechanical ventilation, the principle of autonomy clashes with beneficence. The patient's right to make decisions about their own treatment must be respected, but healthcare providers may struggle with the desire to save the patient's life.

Request for Life-Ending Action: In situations where a competent patient requests the withdrawal of mechanical ventilation, which could lead to their death, the principles of beneficence and autonomy collide once again. Here, the patient's autonomy to make decisions about their own life and death is in direct conflict with the healthcare provider's obligation to do what is best for the patient's well-being.

In conclusion, we need to understand the importance of a nuanced and context-specific approach to ethical decision-making in medicine. Healthcare professionals must carefully weigh the competing ethical principles and make difficult decisions when conflicts arise, always striving to balance the principles of beneficence, non-maleficence, autonomy, and justice in the best interests of the patient. These ethical dilemmas underscore the complexity and moral challenges inherent in the practice of medicine [1, 2].

The concept of beneficence in the context of medical ethics is associated with the potential ethical concerns associated with giving it primacy over patient autonomy, this also includes the concept of paternalism in the physician-patient relationship and distinguishes between soft and hard forms of paternalism. Let us break down each aspect in more detail:

Beneficence in Medicine: Beneficence is one of the fundamental principles of medical ethics, emphasising the obligation of healthcare professionals to act in the best interests of their patients. This principle has a long historical tradition in the practice of medicine. It implies that physicians should aim to provide medical care that promotes the well-being and health of the patient.

Paternalism in Medicine: Paternalism is a term used to describe a situation in which someone in authority (in this case, a physician) makes decisions on behalf of another person (the patient) with the intention of promoting the patient's well-being, even if it means overriding the patient's preferences or autonomy.

Primacy of Beneficence and Paternalism: The passage raises the concern that giving beneficence primacy over patient autonomy can lead to a paternalistic approach in medicine. In a paternalistic relationship, the physician might act like a parent to a child, making decisions for the patient without necessarily involving the patient in the decision-making process. This can include tactics like withholding information, manipulation, deception, or even coercion to steer the patient toward what the physician believes is best.

Soft and Hard Paternalism

Soft Paternalism: This form of paternalism involves actions taken in the best interest of the patient when the patient's capacity to make an informed decision is compromised or when the patient's choice poses a substantial risk to their well-being. Soft paternalism is typically seen as justifiable in situations where the patient's autonomy is limited, such as when they lack decision-making capacity due to mental illness or unconsciousness.

Hard Paternalism: Hard paternalism, on the other hand, involves overriding a patient's autonomous choices even when they are fully informed and competent to make their own decisions. It implies that the physician believes they know better than the patient what is in the patient's best interest and acts accordingly.

While beneficence underscores the importance of doing what is best for the patient, excessive reliance on this principle can lead to paternalistic behaviour in the physician-patient relationship. The extent to which paternalism is ethically justified depends on factors such as the patient's capacity to make decisions and the nature of the medical situation. Soft paternalism is generally considered more acceptable when the patient's autonomy is impaired or when their choices pose significant risks, while hard paternalism, where patient autonomy is disregarded without good reason, is ethically problematic and requires careful consideration in practice [1].

Soft Paternalism

Grounds for Soft Paternalism: Soft paternalism is a form of paternalistic action taken by a physician when the patient is considered non-autonomous or substantially non-autonomous. This lack of autonomy can result from various factors, including cognitive dysfunction due to severe illness, mental health conditions like depression, or addiction to drugs or substances. In such situations, the patient's capacity to make fully informed and rational decisions about their medical care may be compromised.

Ethical Justification: Soft paternalism is ethically justifiable in cases where the patient's autonomy is impaired. The physician's actions are guided by the principles of beneficence (doing what is best for the patient) and, to some extent, non-maleficence (avoiding harm). The underlying assumption is that the patient, if fully autonomous and rational, would likely make a decision consistent with their best interests.

Difficulty in Determination: One of the complexities of soft paternalism lies in determining whether the patient was non-autonomous at the time of decision-making. This retrospective assessment can be challenging, as the patient's mental or emotional state may fluctuate. However, ethically, soft paternalism is considered acceptable as long as the physician's actions align with what they believe to be the patient's values and best interests.

Hard Paternalism

Definition: Hard paternalism involves actions taken by a physician that are intended to benefit a patient but are contrary to the voluntary decision of an autonomous patient who is fully informed and competent. In other words, the patient is capable of making their own decisions, has all the necessary information, and chooses a particular course of action that the physician disagrees with.

Ethical Indefensibility: Hard paternalism is ethically indefensible because it violates the core principle of patient autonomy. In situations where a competent patient makes an informed choice, the physician should respect that choice, even if the physician believes it is not in the patient's best interest. The ethical foundation of medicine is built on respecting a patient's right to self-determination, and hard paternalism disregards this fundamental principle.

Soft paternalism is a nuanced and ethically justifiable approach in situations where a patient's autonomy is compromised due to various factors. It allows the physician to act in the patient's best interests while considering what the patient would likely choose if they were fully autonomous. On the other hand, hard paternalism is ethically problematic because it overrides the autonomy of a competent patient, which is considered a fundamental ethical principle in medical practice. Physicians should always strive to strike a balance between beneficence and patient autonomy, leaning toward paternalism only when it is clearly in the patient's best interests and their autonomy is substantially impaired [1, 3].

The concept of consumerism in healthcare, represents an extreme form of patient autonomy. It contrasts consumerism with hard paternalism and discusses the ethical implications of both approaches. Let us expand on these ideas:

Consumerism in Healthcare

Definition: Consumerism in healthcare is a model where the patient's autonomy and decision-making authority are taken to the extreme. In this model, the physician's role is primarily limited to providing all available medical information and presenting the various choices for interventions and treatments. The fully informed patient is then expected to make decisions independently from these choices.

Patient-Centric Approach: Consumerism places a strong emphasis on patient-centred care, valuing the patient's preferences and choices above all else. It assumes that individuals are best suited to make decisions about their own healthcare, as they are the ones who will ultimately experience the consequences of those decisions.

Limitations on the Physician's Role: In a consumerist model, the physician's role is significantly constrained. They are expected to refrain from making recommendations or guiding the patient's choices beyond providing information. This can limit the physician's ability to use their medical knowledge and expertise to guide patients toward the most appropriate and beneficial treatments.

Ethical Implications of Consumerism

Patient Abandonment: consumerism, when taken to the extreme, can be tantamount to a form of patient abandonment. Patient abandonment occurs when a healthcare provider fails to provide reasonable care to a patient and can have serious ethical and legal consequences. In the context of consumerism, the concern is that physicians may feel obligated to withdraw their expertise and guidance entirely, potentially leaving patients to make complex medical decisions without adequate support.

Ethical Indefensibility: consumerism is ethically indefensible. It raises concerns about whether patients, even when fully informed, are always in the best position to make highly complex medical decisions. It also questions whether the complete withdrawal of the physician's expertise aligns with the physician's ethical duty to act in the best interests of the patient.

Consumerism in healthcare represents a model where patient autonomy is taken to an extreme, with patients being expected to make all medical decisions independently after receiving information from the physician. While patient autonomy is an essential ethical principle in medicine, extreme consumerism can pose challenges and ethical concerns. It can limit the physician's role to such an extent that it may be seen as a form of patient abandonment, raising questions about whether this approach truly serves the best interests of the patient. Striking a balance between patient autonomy and the physician's expertise remains a key challenge in modern healthcare ethics, with different ethical frameworks and models offering varying perspectives on the physician-patient relationship [1, 3].

"Beneficence can be inclusive of patient autonomy as 'the best interests of the patients are intimately linked with their preferences' from which 'are derived our primary duties to them'" highlights the interconnectedness of the principles of beneficence and patient autonomy in the context of medical ethics. Let's elaborate on this concept:

Beneficence and Patient Autonomy

Beneficence: Beneficence is the ethical principle that emphasizes the duty of healthcare providers to act in the best interests of their patients. It involves promoting the well-being and welfare of the patient and making decisions that are likely to benefit them.

Patient Autonomy: Patient autonomy, on the other hand, is the principle that recognizes a patient's right to make informed decisions about their own medical care. It asserts that individuals have the capacity to make choices about their health and medical treatment based on their values, preferences, and goals.

The Interconnectedness of Principles

There is a close relationship between beneficence and patient autonomy. Beneficence can encompass patient autonomy because the best interests of the patient are closely tied to their own preferences and choices.

Patient Preferences and Best Interests: The idea here is that what is genuinely in the best interests of the patient often aligns with their own preferences and values. By respecting the patient's preferences into the decision-making process, healthcare providers are more likely to make choices that genuinely promote the patient's well-being.

Primary Duties to Patients

The primary duties of healthcare providers are derived from the preferences and best interests of the patients. This implies that the ethical obligations of healthcare professionals should be rooted in understanding and respecting the individuality and autonomy of each patient.

Healthcare providers have a duty to consider the patient's values, goals, and preferences when making decisions about their care. By doing so, they are more likely to provide care that is not only medically appropriate but also aligns with the patient's own wishes and desires.

Shared Decision-Making: One practical application of this interconnectedness is shared decision-making. In shared decision-making, healthcare providers collaborate with patients to make decisions about their care. This process recognises the patient's autonomy and preferences while also ensuring that medical expertise is used to provide information and guidance.

Beneficence and patient autonomy are not mutually exclusive principles in medical ethics. Instead, they are intimately linked, with the best interests of the patient often aligning with their own preferences. This understanding underscores the importance of involving patients in their own healthcare decisions and respecting their autonomy as a fundamental aspect of promoting their well-being. Healthcare providers are encouraged to balance these principles by recognising the importance of patient preferences and values when determining the most beneficial course of action for their patients [4].

An important aspect of the physician–patient relationship and the challenges that can arise when there are divergent views on the goals of treatment, especially in evolving medical situations. It underscores the significance of effective communication, particularly when goals of treatment change due to the progression of a disease or other factors. Let's delve deeper into these key points:

Divergent Views on Treatment Goals

Disagreements between physicians and patients regarding treatment are not uncommon. These disagreements often stem from differences in their perceptions of what the goals of treatment should be. Patients may have varying expectations or preferences about the outcomes of their medical care.

Changing Goals of Treatment

As a patient's medical condition evolves, the goals of treatment may also need to change. For example, in chronic neurologic conditions, a patient may eventually require ventilator support, or in cases of refractory cancer, the focus of treatment may shift from curative to palliative care.

Clear and Straightforward Communication

Effective communication is essential in these situations. The physician is encouraged to communicate with the patient in a clear and straightforward manner, avoiding the use of medical jargon or overly technical language that might confuse or intimidate the patient.

Defining New Treatment Goals

When there is a change in the patient's condition, it becomes imperative for the physician to discuss and define the new goals of treatment. This involves a collaborative conversation between the healthcare provider and the patient to ensure a shared understanding of what can be achieved and what the patient values in their care.

Consideration of Decisional Capacity

The physician should be aware of patient factors that can compromise decisional capacity. These factors can include anxiety, fear, pain, lack of trust in the healthcare system or provider, and differences in beliefs and values. Such factors may affect the patient's ability to fully engage in the decision-making process.

Patient-Cenered Approach

In addressing these challenges, a patient-centred approach is essential. This approach places the patient's preferences, values, and goals at the forefront of decision-making. Physicians should listen attentively to the patient's concerns, acknowledge their emotions, and work collaboratively to reach a treatment plan that aligns with the patient's values and what is realistically achievable [5].

The practical application of principles of ethics in clinical practice across various healthcare is very complex. A model presented by Jonsen and colleagues in a resource book for clinicians offers a systematic and widely accepted framework for addressing ethical dilemmas. This framework is structured in a way that aligns with the systematic approach that physicians are trained to use when evaluating and managing medical issues. Let's elaborate on the key aspects of this practical approach to problem-solving in ethics:

Structured Framework

The principles of ethics find practical application through a structured framework for addressing ethical dilemmas. This framework is designed to guide healthcare professionals in a systematic manner when they encounter ethical challenges in their clinical practice.

Model by Jonsen et al.

Jonsen and colleagues have developed a model to help clinicians navigate ethical issues. This model likely incorporates principles such as beneficence, nonmaleficence, autonomy, and justice, which form the foundation of ethical decision-making in medicine.

Logical and Well-Accepted

The model presented by Jonsen and colleagues is described as logical and well-accepted. This implies that it is based on a rational and widely recognised approach to ethical reasoning, making it suitable for practical application in real clinical scenarios.

Systematic Format

This format typically includes components such as the chief complaint, history of present illness, past medical history, pertinent family and social history, review of systems, physical examination, and laboratory and imaging studies. By aligning ethics with this familiar format, healthcare professionals can seamlessly incorporate ethical considerations into their clinical practice.

Problem-Solving in Ethics

The practical approach to problem-solving in ethics involves a step-by-step process for addressing ethical dilemmas. This process likely includes identifying the ethical issue, gathering relevant information, considering the ethical principles at play, evaluating potential courses of action, and making a well-reasoned ethical decision.

Interdisciplinary Collaboration

Ethical problem-solving often requires collaboration among healthcare professionals, including physicians, nurses, ethicists, and other team members. The practical framework likely encourages interdisciplinary discussions to arrive at ethical decisions that are in the best interests of the patient.

This shows us the importance of having a structured and systematic approach to addressing ethical challenges in clinical practice. The model proposed by Jonsen and colleagues serves as a valuable resource for healthcare professionals, helping them navigate complex ethical dilemmas while adhering to recognised ethical principles. This approach ensures that ethical considerations are integrated seamlessly into the decision-making process, ultimately promoting patient-centred care and ethical practice in healthcare settings [6].

The conflict resolution can be summarised as such

Clinical Evaluation: This involves recognising medical issues, exploring available treatment choices, and defining care objectives.

Patient Engagement: It encompasses discovering and clarifying the patient's preferences regarding treatment options and care goals.

Quality of Life (QOL): Consideration of how medical problems, interventions, and treatments impact the patient's QOL, all while being aware of personal biases regarding what constitutes an acceptable QOL.

Contextual Factors: These include a range of factors such as family dynamics, cultural influences, spirituality, religious beliefs, economic considerations, and legal aspects.

By employing this framework, physicians can pinpoint conflicting ethical principles, evaluate and balance them to determine the most appropriate course of action. In instances of uncertainty, they can refer to ethics literature and seek expert opinions for guidance [6].

While patient autonomy is a fundamental ethical principle in healthcare that emphasises an individual's right to make decisions about their own medical treatment based on their values, preferences, and goals. However, there are limitations to patient autonomy in healthcare, which are essential to consider in order to provide safe and ethical care. Here are some key limitations:

Decisional Capacity: Autonomy assumes that the patient has the capacity to make informed decisions. In cases where a patient lacks decisional capacity due to cognitive impairment, mental illness, or other factors, their autonomy may be limited. In such situations, healthcare providers may need to make decisions in the patient's best interests, following legal and ethical guidelines.

Emergency Situations: In emergencies where immediate action is required to save a patient's life or prevent serious harm, there may not be enough time for thorough informed consent. In these cases, healthcare providers may need to act without the patient's explicit consent to provide necessary care.

Children and Minors: Children and minors typically have limited autonomy in healthcare decisions. Parents or legal guardians often make decisions on their behalf. However, as children mature, their autonomy and decision-making capacity may increase, and they may be involved in medical decisions, depending on their age and maturity level.

Coercion and Manipulation: Patients may face external pressure or coercion from family members, cultural or religious beliefs, or even healthcare providers that can limit their ability to make truly autonomous decisions. Recognising and addressing such influences is important in ensuring patient autonomy.

Public Health: In situations where a patient's choices may pose a significant risk to public health, authorities may need to intervene, such as in cases of contagious diseases. Quarantine measures and vaccination requirements are examples of situations where individual autonomy may be restricted for the greater good of public health.

Mental Health: Patients with severe mental illness may experience periods of incapacity, during which their ability to make decisions is impaired. In such cases, decisions about treatment may be made by legal guardians or healthcare providers, following established procedures and guidelines.

Conscientious Objection: Healthcare providers have their own autonomy and may refuse to provide treatments or procedures that go against their deeply held beliefs or values. This can create a conflict between the provider's autonomy and the patient's right to receive certain treatments or services.

Cultural and Religious Beliefs: Patient autonomy can be limited by cultural or religious beliefs that may restrict certain medical interventions or treatments. Balancing respect for these beliefs with the provision of evidence-based care can be challenging.

While patient autonomy is a critical principle in healthcare, there are situations where it may be limited or must be balanced with other ethical principles or legal considerations. Recognising these limitations and navigating complex situations with sensitivity and ethical awareness is essential for providing patient-centred and ethically sound care [5–7].

References

1. Varkey B. Principles of clinical ethics and their application to practice. Med Princ Pract. 2021;30(1):17–28.
2. Beauchamp TL, Childress JF. Principles of bioethics. 7th ed. Oxford University Press; 2013.
3. Tonelli MR, Misak CJ. Compromised autonomy and the seriously ill patient. Chest. 2010;137(4):926–31.
4. Pellegrino E, Thomasma D. For the patient's good: the restoration of beneficence in health care. New York: Oxford University Press; 1988. p. 29.
5. Dubler NN, Liebman CB. Bioethics mediation: a guide to shaping shared solutions. New York, NY: United Hospital Fund of New York; 2004.
6. Jonsen AR, Siegler M, Winslade WJ. Ethics: a practical approach to ethical decisions in clinical medicine. 8th ed. McGraw Hill; 2015.
7. Siegler. CriticalIllness: the limits of autonomy, 7 Hastings Center Rep, 12; 1977.

Chapter 7
Morals and Virtues

Philosophers engaging in moral theory aim to systematise morality. Morality encompasses norms and principles governing human interactions, often considered universal and impartial. Common-sense morality, based on intuitions, guides theory construction. It highlights self/other asymmetries, agent-centred prerogatives, and distinctions like intention vs. foresight. Ethical considerations extend beyond morality, including personal development and projects. Critics find morality too demanding, alienating, and incompatible with special obligations. Some oppose codifiable principles, emphasising agents' responses to the right reasons. Debates explore morality's scope and the role of impartiality. Critics like Bernard Williams argue against moral theory's inescapable obligations and pervasive influence.

Criteria and Moral Theories: Moral philosophy delves into the criteria that guide our judgments about right and wrong actions. Different moral theories provide various criteria for evaluating actions. Here are some key moral theories and their associated criteria:

Consequentialism: The right action is the one that produces the most good among available options.
Kantian Deontology: Morally worthy actions conform to the Categorical Imperative, respecting the rational nature of others.
Rossian Deontology: Right actions align with one's prima facie duties.
Contractualism: Actions are morally wrong if they are forbidden by principles rational persons could not reasonably reject.
Virtue Ethics: The right action reflects what a virtuous person would typically do in the given circumstances.

These principles establish the criteria for assessing actions but don't necessarily prescribe how to perform them. They can be adapted into decision procedures but may require further evaluation based on the specific theory's criteria.

Categorising Moral Theories: Moral theories can be broadly categorised as deontological, consequentialist, or virtue ethical. However, this categorisation can be

S. Abbas, *Medical Ethics*, https://doi.org/10.1007/978-981-96-9199-9_7

debated. Deontological theories focus on duties, consequentialist theories emphasise outcomes, and virtue ethics emphasise character.

Objective and Subjective Standards: Another distinction in moral theories is between objective and subjective standards. Objective standards require the agent to meet the standard to be considered morally right. Subjective standards focus on what the agent believes or could foresee in terms of meeting the standard, considering their psychology or available evidence.

Decision Procedures and Practical Deliberation: Moral theories can serve as decision procedures to guide individuals in making morally right choices. Some view action guidance as the primary function of moral principles. The concept of indirection arises in two forms:

Indirection in Evaluation: For example, Rule Utilitarianism assesses right actions indirectly through rules.

Indirection in Decision Procedures: Sophisticated Consequentialism suggests that explicitly aiming for the right action may not be necessary in all situations. This form acknowledges that other principles or dispositions can align with promoting the good.

The second form relies on the distinction between standards and decision procedures. A middle-ground approach combines self-regulation with periodic consultation of the moral basis for actions.

Moral principles are foundational beliefs and guidelines that shape the ethical framework by which individuals make life choices and decisions. These principles serve as a compass for evaluating the rightness or wrongness of actions and behaviours. Here is how moral principles influence life choices:

Guidance for Decision-Making: Moral principles provide a set of values and norms that help individuals assess and make decisions in various life situations. When faced with ethical dilemmas, individuals turn to their moral principles to determine the morally right course of action.

Consistency in Behaviour: Moral principles promote consistency in behaviour. They encourage individuals to act in ways that align with their deeply held values and beliefs. This consistency contributes to a sense of integrity and moral identity.

Conflict Resolution: Moral principles can help resolve conflicts between competing values and interests. When individuals encounter conflicting priorities, moral principles serve as a framework for weighing and prioritising those values to arrive at a decision.

Personal Growth: Adhering to moral principles can lead to personal growth and character development. It encourages individuals to reflect on their values and make choices that promote moral and ethical growth.

Relationships: Moral principles play a significant role in interpersonal relationships. They guide individuals in treating others with respect, fairness, and empathy. Adherence to these principles fosters healthy and ethical relationships.

Social and Community Impact: Life choices influenced by moral principles have a broader impact on society and communities. They contribute to the development of a just and ethical society by promoting behaviours that respect the rights and well-being of others.

Ethical Dilemmas: Moral principles are especially critical in navigating ethical dilemmas. They help individuals address complex situations where there may be conflicting moral values or obligations, allowing them to make ethically informed choices.

Cultural and Religious Influence: Cultural and religious beliefs often shape an individual's moral principles. These principles reflect the teachings, values, and norms of one's culture or faith tradition and influence a wide range of life choices, from dietary preferences to family values.

Professional Ethics: In professional contexts, individuals often adhere to specific codes of ethics that are rooted in moral principles. These codes guide ethical behaviour in professions such as medicine, law, and business.

Lifelong Moral Journey: Moral principles are not static; they evolve over time as individuals learn, grow, and adapt to changing circumstances. Life choices may be influenced by an evolving understanding of what is morally right and just.

Moral principles serve as the foundation for ethical decision-making and life choices. They guide individuals in living in accordance with their values and beliefs, promoting moral integrity, responsible behaviour, and the well-being of oneself and society as a whole.

The post-medieval revolution in physics and medicine coincided with a profound philosophical shift. A significant figure in this intellectual transformation was the French philosopher René Descartes, also known as Cartesius (1596–1650). Descartes proposed a view that likened all animals to machines, asserting that the human body, like animals, operated as a machine. However, he made a distinctive distinction: the human body was linked to a soul. According to Descartes, souls possessed consciousness and free will, and existed in a temporal dimension but were entirely non-spatial. Remarkably, despite their non-spatial nature, souls could interact with the human body through a specific location called the epiphysis, which was believed to be situated in the pineal gland. In a sense, a soul could permeate and influence its associated body. In the Cartesian perspective, except for actions and events are driven by free will, all internal bodily functions, and externally induced bodily behaviours were to be explicable through mechanisms akin to how machines function. Descartes advocated for explanations rooted in mechanisms, where the motions of certain body parts would cause, or "push," other parts to move in specific ways. Consequently, all notions of teleology, encompassing purposes, goals, and design, were stripped from the body itself. The metaphor of a clockwork swiftly gained popularity as a means to describe and elucidate internal bodily processes. Much like a clock, which serves the externally imposed purpose of indicating time, the body, once created, functioned independently of any externally imposed purpose. Cartesians believed that God had initially designed the human body with a specific purpose in mind. Nonetheless, they argued that the internal functioning of the body should be comprehensively explained through mechanistic principles. It wasn't until the advent of the Darwinian revolution that the concept of a divinely or pre-determined natural design yielded to the purely causal notion of "natural selection" in the realm of biology [1].

Aristotle, the ancient Greek philosopher, introduced the concept of the four cardinal virtues in his ethical philosophy, particularly in his work "Nicomachean Ethics." These virtues are considered fundamental to achieving moral excellence and living a virtuous life according to Aristotle. The four cardinal virtues in Aristotle's philosophy are:

Courage (or Fortitude): In Aristotle's ethical framework, courage, or fortitude, is the virtue that enables individuals to face fear, danger, and adversity with confidence and resolve. It involves the ability to confront difficult situations and act justly, even when facing personal risks. Courage is about finding the right balance between recklessness and cowardice.

Temperance (or Moderation): Temperance is the virtue of self-control and moderation. It involves restraining one's desires and appetites to avoid excesses and maintain a sense of balance and harmony in life. Temperance helps individuals avoid indulgence in pleasures that can lead to moral flaws or harm to themselves and others.

Practical Wisdom (or Prudence): Aristotle referred to practical wisdom as the virtue that enables individuals to make good and morally sound judgments in practical matters. It involves the ability to discern the right course of action in specific situations and to make decisions that align with moral values and virtues. Practical wisdom is about knowing how to apply ethical principles to real-life situations.

Justice: Justice is the virtue that pertains to fairness, equity, and treating others with respect and in accordance with their due. It involves giving each person their rightful share and ensuring that individuals are treated justly and fairly. Justice encompasses both distributive justice (fair distribution of benefits and burdens in society) and rectificatory justice (correcting injustices).

Aristotle believed that these four cardinal virtues represent a balanced and harmonious approach to ethical living. They are interconnected and support one another in the pursuit of moral excellence. For Aristotle, the ultimate goal of human life was "eudaimonia," often translated as "happiness" or "flourishing," which he believed could be achieved through the cultivation of these virtues and the development of a virtuous character.

These four cardinal virtues in Aristotle's ethical philosophy have had a profound influence on Western moral thought and continue to be important concepts in discussions of ethics and virtue ethics [2].

The concept of the "Seven Heavenly Virtues" is a counterpart to the "Seven Deadly Sins" and is often discussed within the context of Christian moral theology. While the Seven Deadly Sins represent negative vices to be avoided, the Seven Heavenly Virtues represent positive virtues to be cultivated. These virtues are seen as virtuous behaviours and attitudes that lead individuals toward spiritual and moral growth. The Seven Heavenly Virtues are:

Chastity: Chastity is the virtue of purity and self-control in matters of sexual desire and behaviour. It encourages individuals to maintain moral and ethical standards in their relationships and to avoid sexual misconduct or impurity.

Temperance: Temperance is the virtue of self-control and moderation in one's desires and appetites. It promotes balance and restraint, helping individuals avoid excesses and maintain a sense of inner harmony.

Charity (or Love): Charity, often referred to as love, is the virtue of selfless love and goodwill toward others. It encourages individuals to show kindness, compassion, and generosity to those in need, both materially and emotionally.

Diligence: Diligence, also known as zeal or industry, is the virtue of commitment, persistence, and hard work. It encourages individuals to exert effort and dedication in their endeavours, pursuing excellence and accomplishing tasks with enthusiasm.

Patience: Patience is the virtue of endurance and tolerance in the face of adversity or difficulties. It promotes the ability to remain calm and composed, even when facing challenges, and to persevere through hardships.

Kindness: Kindness is the virtue of showing empathy, benevolence, and compassion towards others. It encourages acts of goodwill and consideration for the well-being of others, promoting harmonious relationships and a sense of community.

Humility: Humility is the virtue of modesty and self-awareness. It encourages individuals to acknowledge their limitations, recognise their dependence on a higher power, and avoid arrogance or excessive pride.

It is important to note that the Seven Heavenly Virtues are not exclusive to Christianity and can be found in various forms in other moral and philosophical traditions. These virtues are seen as qualities that lead individuals toward spiritual and moral excellence and are often emphasised as part of a virtuous and ethical life.

In both Christianity and Islam, there are theological virtues that play a significant role in the religious and moral lives of believers. These virtues are considered to be divinely infused and are distinct from the cardinal virtues (such as courage, temperance, prudence, and justice) that are acquired through human effort and reason. The three theological virtues shared by both religions are:

Faith (Iman in Islam)

Christianity: In Christianity, faith is the belief in God, the acceptance of Jesus Christ as Lord and Savior, and trust in God's divine plan. It is the foundation of Christian belief and is often described as the assurance of things hoped for and the conviction of things not seen (Hebrews 11:1, New Testament).

Islam: In Islam, Iman (faith) is a central concept. It encompasses belief in the oneness of God (Tawhid), belief in angels, belief in the revealed scriptures (including the Quran and previous divine books), belief in the prophets (including

Muhammad as the final prophet), and belief in the Day of Judgment. Faith is a fundamental pillar of Islamic belief and practice.

Hope (Raja' in Islam)

Christianity: Christian hope is centred on the belief in eternal life with God, often referred to as the hope of salvation. It is the confident expectation of God's promises and the anticipation of a future in God's presence.

Islam: While hope (Raja') is not explicitly labeled as a theological virtue in Islam, it is inherent in the concept of trust in God's mercy and the hope of God's forgiveness. Muslims have hope in God's compassion and mercy, especially on the Day of Judgment.

Charity (Love in Christianity and Ihsan in Islam)

Christianity: In Christianity, the theological virtue of charity is often referred to as love. It is the love of God and the love of neighbor. Christians are called to love one another as Jesus loved them (John 13:34–35, New Testament), and charity is considered one of the greatest virtues (1 Corinthians 13, New Testament).

Islam: In Islam, Ihsan is often equated with charity, but it also encompasses the idea of excellence in one's actions and worship. Charity (Sadaqah) is a fundamental practice in Islam, reflecting generosity, compassion, and care for those in need. The Quran emphasizes the importance of giving to the poor and those less fortunate.

While these theological virtues are shared by Christianity and Islam, their theological interpretations and practices may differ between the two religions. However, the common emphasis on faith, hope, and charity underscores the universal spiritual values that guide the lives of believers in both faith traditions [2].

Aristotle's ethical theories, including his concepts of virtue and the four cardinal virtues, had a significant impact on Western thought and ethics, particularly through the work of scholars like Thomas Aquinas. Here's a brief elaboration on how Aristotle's ideas influenced Aquinas and the broader scholastic tradition:

Incorporation into Scholasticism: Thomas Aquinas, a medieval theologian and philosopher, played a pivotal role in integrating Aristotelian philosophy into Christian theology. Aquinas believed that reason and faith were compatible, and he sought to reconcile Aristotle's philosophical ideas with Christian doctrine.

Virtue Ethics: Aristotle's virtue ethics, which emphasised the cultivation of moral virtues as a means to achieve eudaimonia (flourishing or happiness), resonated with Aquinas. Aquinas incorporated Aristotle's concept of virtue into his ethical framework within the Christian context.

Natural Law Theory: Aquinas developed the natural law theory, which posited that moral principles could be derived from human nature and reason. He believed that by using reason, humans could discern the moral laws inherent in the natural order. This notion was influenced by Aristotle's emphasis on reason and practical wisdom (phronesis).

Four Cardinal Virtues: Aquinas adopted Aristotle's four cardinal virtues (courage, temperance, practical wisdom, and justice) as a foundational framework for moral development and ethical decision-making. These virtues became integral to Thomistic ethics.

Ethical Virtue and Moral Theology: Aquinas integrated Aristotelian virtue ethics with Christian moral theology. He emphasised the importance of cultivating virtues like charity, hope, and faith alongside the cardinal virtues as part of moral and spiritual development.

Ethical Foundations: Aristotle's ethical theories provided a philosophical foundation for Aquinas to address moral questions within a Christian theological framework. The synthesis of Aristotle's philosophy and Christian theology in scholastic thought influenced subsequent discussions of ethics in the Western intellectual tradition.

Overall, the incorporation of Aristotle's ethical ideas, including his concept of virtue and the four cardinal virtues, into the works of Thomas Aquinas and other scholastics played a pivotal role in shaping Western ethical thought and contributed to the development of moral theology within the Catholic Church. These ideas continue to influence contemporary discussions of ethics, virtue ethics, and moral philosophy [3].

The field of medical ethics is relatively recent, emerging towards the close of the eighteenth century. Two distinct responses emerged from eighteenth -century Edinburgh. The initial response was attributed to Thomas Percival, an Edinburgh medical student between 1761 and 1765. He later left to finish his degree at Leyden. Thirty years afterward, Percival had assumed the role of physician at the Manchester Infirmary. He authored medical ethics to establish regulations governing the interactions among healthcare professionals. It served as a blueprint for the self-regulating, paternalistic, and generally benevolent style of professional medical ethics that predominated until approximately the mid-twentieth century. Medical Ethics was a reinterpretation of the Hippocratic principles [4].

A second, very different answer came from John Gregory who published a series of Lectures on the Duties and Qualifications of a Physician. A physician, he believed, had a positive moral duty to be "ready to acknowledge and rectify his mistakes." He contended that the field of medicine would advance more swiftly if physicians practiced "under the supervision and support of individuals qualified to assess their competence and who were not inclined, due to ulterior motives, to undervalue it." Furthermore, this issue was exacerbated by the fact that "the art must be practiced in such a private manner, making it challenging for the public to accurately assess the physician's knowledge based on the success of their practice." He argued that medical practice and knowledge should be open to the public rather than self regulating "the inspection and patronage of men qualified to judge." The superiority of Gregory's solution over Percival's prescription was not fully acknowledged until the mid-twentieth century. That was due to significant biomedical progress in the postwar era, including advancements in in vitro fertilisation and transplant surgery. His approach addressed the question about what medicine should do not what it could do. The changing role of doctors involves relearning effective communication, and sharing both knowledge and uncertainties. The rise of medical ethics as an academic field in the later twentieth century mirrors the evolving dynamics of doctor–patient relationships and the growing significance of informed public participation [5].

References

1. Johansson I, Lynøe N. Medicine & philosophy. A twenty-first century introduction. Ontos Verlag. ISBN 978-3-938793-90-9. p. 1–5.
2. Venard O-T. The belief in the incarnation of god: source of religious humility or cause of theological pride? In: Heft JL, Firestone R, Safi O, editors. Learned ignorance: intellectual humility among Jews, Christians and Muslims. online ed. New York, 2011: Oxford Academic; 2015.
3. Kaczor C, Sherman T. Thomas Aquinas on the cardinal virtues: a summa of the summa on justice, courage, temperance, and practical wisdom. Catholic University of America Press; 2008.
4. Leake CD, editor. Percival's medical ethics. Huntington, NY: Robert E Kreiger Publishing Company; 1975.
5. Gregory J. The duties and qualifications of a physician. In: Broadie A, editor. The Scottish enlightenment: an anthology. Edinburgh: Canongate; 1997. 760ff.

Chapter 8
Human Rights

The power of the Universal Declaration is the power of ideas to change the world. It inspires us to continue working to ensure all people can gain freedom, equality and dignity.

It is a controversial issue to consider healthcare as an essential human right, some have argued, that access to healthcare should be considered a fundamental human right because it is a crucial prerequisite for leading a fulfilling life. He presents his argument for this perspective as follows:

All individuals possess human rights to the fundamental conditions necessary for the pursuit of a fulfilling life.
Fundamental health is among these necessary conditions for the pursuit of a fulfilling life.

Therefore, all individuals possess a human right to fundamental health.

A human right to fundamental health entails a human right to the indispensable resources required for preserving and advancing fundamental health.

Fundamental healthcare represents one of these indispensable resources for preserving and advancing fundamental health.

Consequently, there exists a human right to fundamental healthcare [1].

Human rights are fundamental principles and entitlements that apply to all individuals, regardless of their nationality, ethnicity, gender, religion, or any other characteristic. They are considered inherent to human beings and are designed to protect and promote the dignity, freedom, and well-being of every person. Here are the basics of human rights:

Universal and Inalienable: Human rights are universal, meaning they apply to all people in all places at all times. They are inalienable, which means they cannot be taken away or surrendered, even by an individual's consent.
Interconnected and Interdependent: Human rights are interconnected and interdependent. This means that the enjoyment of one right often depends on the fulfilment of other rights. For example, the right to education can be realised more

S. Abbas, *Medical Ethics*, https://doi.org/10.1007/978-981-96-9199-9_8

effectively when there is access to health care and freedom from discrimination.

Inherent Dignity: Human rights are based on the inherent dignity of every human being. They recognise that each person has intrinsic worth and should be treated with respect and without discrimination.

Civil, Political, Economic, Social, and Cultural Rights: Human rights are typically categorised into different types, including civil and political rights (e.g., the right to life, freedom of speech), and economic, social, and cultural rights (e.g., the right to education, health care). Both sets of rights are essential for a person's well-being.

Legal Protection: Human rights are often protected by national and international laws. Many countries have laws and constitutions that explicitly recognise and protect human rights. Additionally, international treaties and agreements, such as the Universal Declaration of Human Rights and the International Covenant on Civil and Political Rights, provide a framework for safeguarding human rights globally.

Equality and Non-Discrimination: Human rights promote equality and non-discrimination. They prohibit discrimination on the basis of race, colour, sex, religion, national or social origin, disability, and other factors. All individuals should have equal access to their human rights.

Government Responsibility: Governments have a primary responsibility to respect, protect, and fulfil human rights within their jurisdictions. This includes refraining from violating rights, preventing violations by others, and taking proactive steps to ensure that people can enjoy their rights.

Accountability and Remedies: When human rights are violated, individuals have the right to seek justice and remedies. This may involve legal action, advocacy, or other means to hold perpetrators accountable and obtain redress for harm suffered.

Civil Society and Advocacy: Civil society organisations, activists, and advocacy groups play a crucial role in promoting and defending human rights. They raise awareness, advocate for policy changes, and hold governments and institutions accountable for upholding human rights.

Ongoing Challenges: Despite significant progress in recognising and protecting human rights, challenges persist worldwide. Issues such as discrimination, poverty, conflict, and violations of political freedoms continue to be areas of concern that require ongoing attention and action.

Human rights provide a framework for a just and fair society, where individuals are able to live with dignity, freedom, and equality. They are a fundamental part of international law and ethical principles and are essential for promoting peace, justice, and human development worldwide [2].

It is important to refer to Article 25 of the Universal Human Declaration:

Everyone has the right to a standard of living adequate for the health and well-being of himself and his family, including food, clothing, housing and medical care and necessary social services, and the right to security in the event of unemployment, sickness, disability, widowhood, old age or other lack of livelihood in circumstances beyond his control.

Motherhood and childhood are entitled to special care and assistance. All children, whether born in or out of wedlock, shall enjoy the same social protection [3].

Everyone has the right to a standard of living adequate for the health and well-being of himself and his family, including food, clothing, housing and medical care and necessary social services, and the right to security in the event of unemployment, sickness, disability, widowhood, old age or other lack of livelihood in circumstances beyond his control.

Motherhood and childhood are entitled to special care and assistance. All children, whether born in or out of wedlock, shall enjoy the same social protection. The question of whether healthcare is an essential human right is a matter of ongoing debate and varies depending on cultural, political, and ethical perspectives. However, many international organisations, medical professionals, and human rights advocates argue that healthcare is indeed an essential human right. Here are some reasons why healthcare is often considered a fundamental human right:

Right to Life and Dignity: Healthcare is closely tied to the right to life and the preservation of human dignity. Access to healthcare services, including preventive care, treatment, and medical interventions, can often be a matter of life and death. Protecting and preserving human life is a fundamental ethical and moral principle.

Universal Declaration of Human Rights: The Universal Declaration of Human Rights, adopted by the United Nations in 1948, recognises the right to healthcare. Article 25 of the declaration states that "everyone has the right to a standard of living adequate for the health and well-being of himself and of his family, including food, clothing, housing, and medical care."

International Human Rights Agreements: Several international human rights agreements and treaties, such as the International Covenant on Economic, Social and Cultural Rights, affirm the right to the highest attainable standard of health. These agreements place an obligation on governments to ensure access to healthcare services for their populations.

Promotion of Equality and Non-Discrimination: Ensuring access to healthcare promotes equality and non-discrimination. Denying healthcare based on factors such as race, gender, socioeconomic status, or disability is considered a violation of human rights principles.

Preventing Suffering and Disability: Access to healthcare can prevent unnecessary suffering and disability. It addresses not only physical health but also mental health, ensuring that individuals can live free from pain, illness, and the debilitating effects of untreated conditions.

Economic and Social Development: Good health is essential for personal well-being and economic productivity. Access to healthcare contributes to economic and social development by allowing individuals to lead healthy and productive lives, reducing the economic burden of disease, and enhancing overall societal well-being.

Ethical Imperative: Many ethical and philosophical perspectives argue for the provision of healthcare as a moral imperative. Ethical frameworks, such as utilitarianism or principles of justice, often support the idea that healthcare should be available to all, especially to those in need.

Public Health and Pandemic Preparedness: Public health measures, including healthcare access, are vital for the well-being of communities and nations. Ensuring access to healthcare is critical in responding to public health crises, such as pandemics, and in preventing the spread of disease.

While there is a strong argument for healthcare as a fundamental human right, the extent to which this right is realised can vary greatly among countries and regions. Access to healthcare services, quality of care, and the financing of healthcare systems are complex issues that continue to be a focus of policy debates and efforts to improve healthcare equity and access worldwide [4, 5].

Common misconceptions about the right to health include thinking it guarantees good health (it is about access to conditions for health) and that it's only a long-term goal (immediate obligations exist). A country's financial situation doesn't absolve it from taking action; states must work toward realising the right to health within their available resources [3–6].

The Committee on Economic, Social and Cultural Rights, is the body responsible for monitoring the International Covenant on Economic, Social and Cultural Rights. The right to health is an inclusive right, encompassing factors beyond just access to healthcare, such as safe drinking water, nutrition, and gender equality. It includes freedoms like protection from non-consensual medical treatment and torture. It also entails entitlements such as access to healthcare services and essential medicines. Health services must be provided without discrimination and must be available, accessible, acceptable, and of good quality [7, 8].

References

1. Liao M. Health (care) and human rights: a fundamental conditions approach. Theor Med Bioeth. 2016;
2. UN. International covenant on economic, social and cultural rights (ICESCR). GA Res. 1966;2200A(XXI):12.
3. https://www.ohchr.org/en/human-rights/universal-declaration/translations/english
4. https://www.who.int/news-room/commentaries/detail/health-is-a-fundamental-human-right
5. See Vienna Declaration and Programme of Action (A/CONF.157/23), adopted by the World Conference on Human Rights, held in Vienna, 14–25 June 1993.
6. The Covenant was adopted by the United Nations General Assembly in its resolution 2200A (XXI) of 16 December 1966. It entered into force in 1976 and by 1 December 2007 had been ratified by 157 States.
7. Nampewo Z, Mike JH, Wolff J. Respecting, protecting and fulfilling the human right to health. Int J Equity Health. 2022;21:36.
8. UN Committee on Economic, Social, and Cultural Rights. General Comment no. 14 the Right to the Highest Attainable Standard of Health (Article 12 of the International Covenant on Economic, Social, and Cultural Rights). Aug 11, 2000, E/C.12/2000/4.

Chapter 9
When Autonomy Undermines Equity

In Western societies, patient autonomy has become the norm However, a series of experiments involving over 3800 participants reveals that when people face complex decisions, they actually prefer guidance and a more paternalistic approach, contrary to the prevailing trend of autonomy. Surprisingly, those providing advice often underestimate this preference for paternalism, resulting in perceptions of lower competence and helpfulness. This preference holds true across various contexts with expert-non-expert dynamics, both in and outside of the medical field. Ultimately, this challenges the recent emphasis on full decisional autonomy in medical care and decision-making.

Suppose you're recently diagnosed with a serious illness and faced with a challenging choice between two options for treatments each with their own pros and cons. Despite having all the information from your doctor, you're still unsure about the best option. In this situation, your doctor would review the costs and benefits, acknowledging that there's no one-size-fits-all answer. They might share what other patients have chosen and their preferences but stress the uncertainty of the outcomes. Your doctor encourages you to weigh your own preferences based on the information provided and make your own decision. Hence, a doctor who prioritises patient-driven decision-making might avoid explicitly suggesting a particular course of action guided by their personal preferences, as they are concerned that such a recommendation could be seen as paternalistic [1, 2].

In situations where there's no clear-cut answer regarding the best course of action for a patient due to uncertainty, patients may defer to the doctor's recommendation rather than relying on their own preferences. This could give the doctor's explicit recommendation an unintended coercive effect [2].

S. Abbas, *Medical Ethics*, https://doi.org/10.1007/978-981-96-9199-9_9

References

1. Schneider C. The practice of autonomy: patients, doctors, and medical decisions. Oxford, UK: Oxford University; 1998.
2. Scherr KA, et al. Physician recommendations trump patient preferences in prostate cancer treatment decisions. Med Decision Making. 2017;37:56–69.

Chapter 10
Justice

Justice is a complex and multifaceted concept that plays a central role in our understanding of fairness and ethical decision-making. It can take on different meanings in various practical contexts, encompassing a wide range of concerns related to how individuals are treated and their rightful claims to fundamental aspects of life, such as freedom, opportunities, and resources.

One of the fundamental distinctions within the realm of justice is its differentiation from charity and mercy. Justice is not solely about acts of benevolence or kindness; it is about upholding and protecting individual rights and entitlements. Unlike charity, which involves discretionary acts of goodwill, justice entails the recognition and enforcement of rights, and it often takes precedence over considerations like economic efficiency or environmental value in shaping public policies and legal frameworks.

Justice operates on several levels, each with its own characteristics:

Individual Claims: At its core, justice involves individuals making claims to assert their rights and resolve conflicts. When people appeal to justice, they seek a fair determination of what they are entitled to. Justice provides a framework for adjudicating these conflicting claims, ensuring that each person receives their due.

Enforceable Obligations: Justice goes beyond abstract principles and involves enforceable obligations. It requires responsible agents, whether individuals or institutions, to take action and alter circumstances to rectify injustices or protect rights. This may involve legal sanctions, compensation, or redistributive measures.

Impartial and Consistent Application: Justice demands the impartial and consistent application of rules and principles. It strives to treat individuals fairly and equally, regardless of personal characteristics or circumstances, and seeks to avoid arbitrary or discriminatory decisions.

Furthermore, there are four key distinctions within the concept of justice:

S. Abbas, *Medical Ethics*, https://doi.org/10.1007/978-981-96-9199-9_10

Conservative vs. Ideal Justice: Justice can be conservative, where it upholds existing norms and practices, or it can be idealistic, demanding reform and the creation of new entitlements and expectations. Conservative justice maintains the status quo, while ideal justice seeks to improve and reshape societal norms.

Corrective vs. Distributive Justice: Corrective justice focuses on remedying wrongs when one person interferes with another's legitimate holdings or rights. In contrast, distributive justice concentrates on the equitable allocation of resources and opportunities among individuals within society.

Procedural vs. Substantive Justice: Procedural justice concerns the fairness of the procedures used to determine outcomes. It emphasises due process and ensuring that decision-making methods are unbiased and transparent. Substantive justice, on the other hand, pertains to the justice of the final allocation itself, regardless of the process.

Comparative vs. Non-Comparative Justice: Justice can be comparative when it involves making comparisons between individuals' claims or outcomes. Alternatively, it can be non-comparative, where claims are determined based on individual characteristics or needs, rather than in relation to others.

The scope of justice is also a matter of inquiry, as it raises questions about when and among whom principles of justice apply. While some principles of justice are universal and apply to all individuals, others may be contextual, relevant only within specific social, political, or institutional relationships.

In conclusion, justice is a multifaceted and dynamic concept that requires careful consideration in various practical and ethical contexts. It is concerned with fundamental questions of fairness, rights, and obligations, and it plays a crucial role in shaping our moral and legal frameworks. Understanding the different dimensions and distinctions within justice is essential for addressing complex ethical issues and advancing social and political discourse [1].

"Justice for Animals" addresses the ethical and philosophical questions surrounding the moral consideration and rights of non-human animals. Historically, many philosophers excluded animals from the realm of justice, but there is a growing advocacy for extending justice to animals in contemporary discourse.

The criteria for determining whether a creature deserves justice are a subject of debate. John Rawls, a prominent philosopher, argues that animals fall outside the scope of justice because they lack the moral capacities necessary for participating in cooperative ventures for mutual advantage. According to Rawls, justice involves reciprocity, which he believes animals cannot engage in. However, this viewpoint is challenged by those who argue for "justice for animals." Advocates for animal justice emphasise non-comparative principles, focusing on the rights of animals against cruelty and ensuring they have basic necessities like food and shelter.

The debate also extends to whether justice should be relational or non-relational. Relational justice is concerned with specific relationships among individuals or groups, while non-relational justice has a broader scope. Rawlsian views suggest that justice arises within cooperative practices, while other theories tie it to citizenship within a state. This debate has significant implications for discussions on global inequality and social justice, as it pertains to whether distributive justice should be considered on a global scale or limited to specific groups or societies.

The question of whether individuals or institutions are responsible for delivering justice is another important consideration. In a society where institutions are established to uphold justice, individuals must grapple with their duties. Should individuals merely support these institutions, or should they actively promote justice in their daily lives? This question often arises in scenarios involving parents granting advantages to their children or wage differentials based on bargaining power. The distinction between principles of justice that apply to societal rules and those that guide personal behaviour underscores the complexity of the scope of justice.

Recent philosophical discussions have also highlighted the concept of justice beyond material treatment, emphasising recognition and identity. Recognition theorists argue that justice encompasses being adequately and appropriately recognised, extending beyond material distribution. Epistemic injustices, such as testimonial injustice and hermeneutic injustice, explore how recognition intersects with knowledge and identity. The relationship between recognition-based justice and distributive justice remains a topic of ongoing debate.

Utilitarianism, a consequentialist ethical theory, seeks to accommodate and explain common intuitions about justice. However, it faces challenges in aligning justice with the maximisation of utility. Prominent utilitarians like John Stuart Mill and Henry Sidgwick have explored the relationship between utility and justice. Mill argues that justice is of paramount importance to human well-being and suggests that it represents a matter of perfect obligation. Sidgwick connects justice to moral emotions like resentment and gratitude, further delving into the distinctiveness of justice within the utilitarian framework.

In summary, the concept of justice is a multifaceted and evolving area of philosophical inquiry, encompassing debates about its application to animals, the relational or non-relational nature of justice, the roles of individuals and institutions, the importance of recognition in justice, and its relationship with utilitarianism. These discussions reflect the ongoing quest to define and understand justice in the context of complex ethical and societal challenges [2].

Utilitarian theories of justice encounter three significant challenges that have prompted philosophical exploration of alternative approaches:

Focus on Distribution vs. Subjective Happiness: Utilitarianism is primarily concerned with maximising overall happiness or utility. However, justice, as commonly understood, places a distinct emphasis on the fair distribution of tangible benefits and burdens among individuals. Justice involves determining rights, opportunities, and entitlements based on principled considerations, rather than relying on the subjective happiness or unhappiness of individuals. This division of labor in ethical theory means that utilitarianism deals with aggregating individual utilities but does not directly address how these utilities translate into principles of fairness. The conversion of principles of justice into units of utility is left to each recipient, and this can raise questions about the fairness of outcomes.

Neglect of Distribution Within Utility: Utilitarianism's focus on maximising overall utility can sometimes disregard how that utility is distributed among individuals. This can lead to morally problematic conclusions, such as the prioritisation of the interests of a "utility monster"—an individual whose utility gains far outweigh others, potentially at the expense of justice. This situation contradicts common intuitions about fairness and equity, as it appears to justify favouring one individual's utility at the cost of others.

Consequentialist Nature vs. Intrinsic Properties: Utilitarianism is a consequentialist ethical theory that evaluates actions and rules solely based on their outcomes in terms of utility. This perspective tends to overlook intrinsic properties or backward-looking reasons related to deservingness or entitlement, which are often central to our understanding of justice. Justice frequently involves considerations of past actions, historical entitlements, and principles that transcend mere utility calculations. Utilitarianism's failure to capture the moral significance of justice in this regard can be seen as a limitation.

In response to these challenges, some philosophers have turned to contractarian and egalitarian theories of justice as alternatives:

Contractarian Theories: Contractarian theories propose that justice emerges from a hypothetical agreement among rational individuals who deliberate on principles for governing institutions and behaviour. Unlike utilitarianism, which aims to maximise overall utility, contractarian theories ensure that principles are chosen to prevent outcomes that individuals would find unacceptable. This approach places an emphasis on fairness and consensus rather than aggregate happiness. John Rawls' contractarian theory, in particular, introduces the concept of the "original position," where decision-makers are situated behind a "veil of ignorance" regarding their own personal characteristics. This veil of ignorance leads to the selection of principles that prioritise equal basic liberties and the well-being of the least advantaged, reflecting a concern for distributive justice and fairness.

While utilitarianism offers a consequentialist framework focused on overall utility, it faces challenges in addressing the distribution of benefits, potential tyranny of the utility monster, and the neglect of intrinsic aspects of justice. Contractarian and egalitarian theories of justice, such as Rawls' original position, offer alternative approaches that emphasise fairness, consensus, and distributive justice as ways to address these challenges and provide a more comprehensive account of justice [3, 4].

T.M. Scanlon's contractarianism focuses on principles that people cannot reasonably reject as a basis for informed, unforced general agreement. This approach allows for some level of inequality when it is justifiable based on the well-being of others.

Egalitarian theories of justice assert that justice often requires substantive equality, especially when there are no distinguishing features among individuals or when we lack information to measure relevant claims to resources or benefits. One approach involves considering characteristics as "morally arbitrary" and discounting claims of desert based on those characteristics. Another approach emphasises the value of equal concern and respect for persons, which can sometimes justify equal treatment even in the presence of relevant differences.

In summary, utilitarian theories of justice face challenges related to the focus on utility, while contractarian and egalitarian theories offer alternative approaches to address these concerns and provide a more robust account of justice [5, 6].

Responsibility-sensitive egalitarianism responds to the objection that simple equality of treatment does not account for individual agency and choices. It allows for deviations from equal distribution when these result from responsible decisions made by individuals. Various versions of this theory, such as luck egalitarianism, differ in their criteria for responsibility, the baseline of equality, and which consequences of choices are considered just. Luck egalitarians argue that inequalities arising from "brute" bad luck should be rectified, while those resulting from responsible choices are permissible. However, this view faces challenges in assessing responsibility and accounting for the influence of innate traits on choices [6, 7].

Relational egalitarianism is a philosophical perspective that places a significant emphasis on social equality within a society. While it doesn't offer a direct and comprehensive theory of justice like some other philosophical approaches, it provides compelling reasons for limiting material inequality based on its core idea: that a divided society with large income disparities can hinder mutual respect and interaction among its members.

Here are key points to elaborate on this concept:

Social Equality as a Central Concern: Relational egalitarianism is primarily concerned with how individuals treat each other as equals within the social fabric of a community or society. It underscores the importance of fostering an environment in which all members regard and interact with each other as social equals.

Not a Comprehensive Theory of Justice: Unlike some other theories of justice, such as utilitarianism or John Rawls' contractarianism, relational egalitarianism does not provide a fully developed and detailed theory of justice with specific principles or rules. Instead, it operates as a lens through which to view the consequences of material inequality and social division.

Limiting Material Inequality: Relational egalitarianism suggests that large income disparities and significant material inequalities can undermine the sense of social equality. When some members of society possess vastly more wealth and resources than others, it can lead to disparities in power, access to opportunities, and influence over decision-making processes. These disparities, in turn, can erode the sense of mutual respect and equal treatment among individuals.

Importance of Mutual Respect and Interaction: The underlying assumption of relational egalitarianism is that a society in which individuals respect each other as equals and interact with mutual respect is more desirable and just. Material inequality can lead to social hierarchies and divisions, making it difficult for individuals from different economic strata to engage with each other as equals.

Conclusion on the Nature of Justice

The concept of justice is multifaceted and can take on different meanings depending on the context in which it is applied. Three overarching frameworks—utilitarianism, contractarianism, and egalitarianism—have been explored as attempts to capture the essence of justice. However, each of these frameworks has its limitations and may not fully encompass the diverse and evolving beliefs about justice held by individuals and societies.

The study of the historical evolution of the concept of justice can provide valuable insights into its variations and how these variations relate to changing societal structures, norms, and values. By examining the historical development of ideas about justice, we can better understand how different societies have grappled with questions of fairness, distribution, and the principles that should govern their interactions. This historical perspective can enrich our understanding of justice and inform contemporary debates about what justice requires in various domains of human life [8–11].

Balancing Access, Equity, and Ethical Dilemmas

Justice in healthcare is a complex and multifaceted concept that revolves around the fair and equitable distribution of healthcare resources, services, and opportunities. It encompasses ethical, social, and economic considerations and plays a crucial role in healthcare policy, medical ethics, and public discourse. Several key aspects define the concept of justice in healthcare:

Access to Healthcare

Universal Healthcare: Many societies strive for universal healthcare, aiming to ensure that every individual, regardless of their socioeconomic status, has access to essential healthcare services. Achieving universal healthcare is often considered a fundamental principle of justice in healthcare.

Healthcare Disparities: Justice requires addressing healthcare disparities that result from factors such as income, race, ethnicity, gender, geography, and disability. Reducing these disparities is essential for creating a more just healthcare system.

Resource Allocation

Equitable Distribution: Distributing healthcare resources, such as medical facilities, healthcare professionals, and medical treatments, equitably is a central concern. Justice in healthcare demands that resources are allocated in a way that addresses the needs of various populations, especially vulnerable or underserved groups.

Priority Setting: Healthcare systems often face limitations in resources, leading to difficult decisions about resource allocation. Ethical frameworks like utilitarianism, egalitarianism, and the capability approach are applied to determine how to prioritise care and allocate scarce resources fairly.

Ethical Dilemmas

Resource Scarcity: The allocation of scarce resources, such as organ transplants or ventilators during a pandemic, presents ethical dilemmas. Decisions must balance the principles of maximising benefits, treating individuals fairly, and respecting autonomy.

End-of-Life Care: Determining when and how to provide or withhold life-sustaining treatments, like life support or palliative care, raises questions of justice, autonomy, and the best interests of the patient.

Healthcare Financing

Health Insurance: Ensuring that individuals have access to health insurance is seen as a matter of justice. The absence of health coverage can result in financial barriers to healthcare and unequal access.

Affordability: Healthcare costs must be affordable for all individuals. High medical expenses can lead to financial hardship, reinforcing health disparities.

Ethical Frameworks

Principles of Medical Ethics: The principles of medical ethics, including beneficence, non-maleficence, autonomy, and justice, guide healthcare professionals in their decision-making. Justice, in this context, relates to treating patients fairly and without discrimination.

Rights-Based Approaches: Some argue that justice in healthcare involves recognising healthcare as a human right. This perspective places a moral obligation on societies to ensure equitable access to healthcare services.

Healthcare Policy

Legislation and Regulation: Government policies and regulations, such as the Affordable Care Act (ACA) in the United States or national healthcare systems in many other countries, are designed to promote justice by expanding access to healthcare services and addressing disparities.

Health Equity Initiatives: Healthcare organisations and policymakers often implement programs and initiatives aimed at reducing health disparities and promoting health equity, aligning with principles of justice.

In conclusion, justice in healthcare is a multifaceted concept that revolves around ensuring equitable access to healthcare services, addressing disparities, making ethically sound decisions in resource allocation, and promoting the well-being of all individuals. Achieving justice in healthcare requires ongoing efforts in healthcare policy, ethics, and practice to create a healthcare system that prioritises fairness, equality, and ethical principle [12, 13].

An argument for justice might be that cancer patients are given priority treatment, and this makes other people's healthcare easier to access. A counter-argument might be that this means other services get less funding. Another argument might be that spending public money on radio- and chemotherapy is cheaper than other treatments. A counter-argument would be that early treatment increases survival rates and actually reduces the cost of cancer treatment.

Priority Treatment for Cancer Patients

Argument: Prioritising cancer patients for treatment can be seen as a just approach because it addresses a pressing medical need. Cancer is a life-threatening disease, and providing prompt care to those diagnosed can improve their chances of survival and quality of life. By allocating resources to cancer treatment, healthcare systems demonstrate their commitment to addressing severe health conditions promptly.

Counter-Argument: While prioritising cancer treatment may seem just, it can have unintended consequences. Allocating a significant portion of healthcare resources to cancer care may mean that resources are diverted away from other medical services. This can lead to longer waiting times for non-cancer patients, potentially harming their health outcomes. Critics argue that a more balanced allocation of resources is needed to ensure fairness and access for all patients, not just those with cancer.

Argument 2: Cost-Effectiveness of Radio- and Chemotherapy

Argument: Another argument for prioritising cancer treatment, particularly radio- and chemotherapy, is that it can be cost-effective in the long run. These treatments, when administered early, can effectively manage cancer, prevent its progression, and potentially lead to a cure. In comparison to late-stage cancer treatment or palliative care, early interventions like chemotherapy may be less expensive for the healthcare system overall.

Counter-Argument: While radio- and chemotherapy can be cost-effective, focusing solely on these treatments neglects the economic benefits of early cancer detection and prevention. Critics argue that investing in preventive measures, such as cancer screenings and public health campaigns, can reduce the incidence of cancer cases, lowering the overall financial burden on the healthcare system. Additionally, early detection often leads to less aggressive treatment, reducing the physical and financial toll on patients and the healthcare system.

Counter-Argument 2: Resource Allocation and Early Treatment

Argument: Early treatment for cancer patients can be seen as justifiable because it reduces the long-term financial burden of cancer care on the healthcare system. Early detection and treatment often lead to higher survival rates, shorter hospital stays, and less aggressive interventions, all of which can lower the overall cost of cancer treatment.

Counter-Argument: While early treatment may reduce long-term costs, it does not eliminate the need for significant upfront investments in diagnostic tools, cancer screenings, and preventive measures. Critics argue that reallocating resources from early detection and prevention to immediate treatment may lead to an increased incidence of cancer cases, ultimately straining the healthcare system's budget in the long run. Moreover, focusing solely on cost savings may compromise the principle of justice by potentially excluding individuals from early detection programs.

In summary, the debate surrounding the prioritisation of cancer treatment revolves around balancing the immediate needs of cancer patients with the long-term sustainability of healthcare systems. Arguments in favour of priority treatment emphasise the severity of the disease and potential cost savings, while counter-arguments highlight the importance of resource allocation, early detection, and preventive measures to ensure equitable and sustainable healthcare access for all [14, 15].

In the realm of healthcare rationing decisions, three primary categories of justice principles are frequently proposed in academic discourse: need principles, maximisation principles, and egalitarian principles. However, each of these principles exhibits a narrower focus compared to the pluralistic combination of principles that seem to garner support from the general public. Philosophers have yet to construct a comprehensive theory that effectively integrates all three of these principles into a coherent framework [15, 16].

One possible explanation for the absence of such a theory in philosophical discourse is that philosophers might not view aligning with public opinion as their primary objective. Instead, they may perceive their role as one of identifying errors and clarifying misconceptions within prevailing public thought. In essence, the public's attempt to amalgamate such a pluralistic set of rationing principles could be seen as misguided or confused.

Alternatively, philosophers may have been hesitant to delve into the subject of justice in healthcare rationing decisions altogether. Much of the literature on this topic, although not exclusively, is penned by health economists. Philosophers with expertise in medical ethics often concentrate on decisions concerning individual patients rather than the equitable allocation of healthcare resources among patients. Those specialising in moral and political philosophy, in a broader context, tend to focus on foundational decisions related to the fundamental institutions of the healthcare system, as opposed to the day-to-day policy decisions that govern its operation.

This reluctance among professional philosophers to engage with the practical policy questions surrounding justice in healthcare rationing is evident in the works of scholars like Daniels, who expands upon Rawls's renowned theory of justice to apply it to the healthcare system. Daniels advocates a comprehensive theory suggesting that the healthcare system should be designed to bring every individual as close as possible to a minimum threshold of health, termed "normal species functioning." However, he acknowledges that policymakers may not find immediate answers to their pressing questions within this theoretical framework. Similarly, Richard Hare, who endorses an advanced utilitarian theory and applies it to various issues in applied ethics, admits his limited expertise when it comes to healthcare. He states, "I am not very well versed in the details of these problems, and have had to content myself with giving what I think is the best philosophical basis for their solution, leaving it to others to apply it to the various difficulties that all who seek to provide an adequate health service are faced with."

There exists significant potential for further philosophical exploration aimed at constructing new theories of justice in healthcare rationing that embrace a more pluralistic approach than simply relying on need-based distribution or health maximisation. These theories should strive to align more closely with the moral intuitions held by the general public [15–18].

References

1. Aristotle. Nicomachean ethics, trans by Roger Crisp. Cambridge: Cambridge University Press; 2000.
2. Bentham J. The principles of morals and legislation. Laurence Lafleur, New York: Hafner Press; 1948.

3. Cohen GA. On the currency of egalitarian justice. Ethics. 1989;99:906–44.
4. Donaldson S, Kymlicka W. Zoopolis: a political theory of animals rights. Oxford: Oxford University Press; 2011.
5. Fleischacker S. A short history of distributive justice. Cambridge, MA: Harvard University Press; 2004.
6. Fraser N, Honneth A. Redistribution or recognition? : A political-philosophical exchange. London: Verso; 2003.
7. Mill JS. Utilitarianism. In: Lindsay AD, editor. Utilitarianism, on liberty, representative government. London: Dent; 1964.
8. Nozick R. Anarchy, State and Utopia. Oxford: Blackwell; 1974.
9. Sandel M. Liberalism and the limits of justice. Cambridge: Cambridge University Press; 1982.
10. Scanlon TM. What we owe to each other. Cambridge, MA: Harvard University Press; 1998.
11. Sidgwick H. The methods of ethics. London: Macmillan; 1874/1907.
12. Beauchamp TL, Childress JF. Principles of biomedical ethics. Oxford: Oxford University Press; 1979.
13. Cookson R, Dolan P. Public views on health care rationing: a group discussion study. Health Policy. 1999;49:63–74.
14. Culyer AJ. The principle objective of the NHS should be to maximise aggregate health. In: New B, editor. Rationing: talk and action in health care. London: King's Fund and British Medical Journal Publishing Group; 1997.
15. Broome J. Good, fairness and QALYs. In: Bell M, Mendus S, editors. Philosophy and medical welfare. Cambridge: University of Cambridge Press; 1988.
16. Williams A. Intergenerational equity: an exploration of the 'fair innings' argument. Health Econ. 1997;6(2):117–32.
17. Rawls J. A theory of justice. Cambridge, MA: Harvard University Press; 1971.
18. Hare R. Health care policy: some options. In: Hare R, editor. Essays on bioethics. Oxford: Clarendon Press; 1993. p. 209–18.

Chapter 11
Health Care Rationing

There is a suggestion that there is an opportunity for more research by philosophers and social scientists to create a comprehensive and diverse theory of healthcare rationing that aligns with public opinion. This chapter delves into the fourth principle ethics: in the realm of daily healthcare priority-setting or rationing decisions made by clinicians and administrators, what is the true essence of "justice"?

The academic literature commonly explores three justice principles in healthcare rationing decisions: need principles, maximising principles, and egalitarian principles. This chapter conducts a comparison and contrast of these three principles in the context of a hypothetical rationing dilemma in order to elucidate the similarities and differences inherent in each principle. The primary rationing principles derived from the literature can be categorised into three major groups: need principles, maximising principles, and egalitarian principles. Need principles advocate for healthcare distribution based on "need," such as immediate ill health. Maximising principles advocate for healthcare distribution to achieve the maximum "benefit," focusing on population health. Lastly, egalitarian principles advocate for healthcare distribution to reduce "inequality," considering factors like lifetime health [1]. Each of these principles has a narrower focus compared to the pluralistic combination supported by the general public. Philosophers have not yet developed a coherent theory that integrates all three principles.

The Need Principle

Allocating healthcare based on need is a highly debated rationing principle, extensively discussed in both academic and non-academic discussions. Clinicians, who perceive themselves as expert evaluators of need, commonly employ the term "clinical need." This principle is notably favoured and prevalent in debates. Nevertheless, without a precise definition of "clinical need" incorporating substantive criteria, this principle devolves into a less appealing procedural notion, implying that any

S. Abbas, *Medical Ethics*, https://doi.org/10.1007/978-981-96-9199-9_11

rationing decision is deemed correct as long as a clinician has made it, Distinct interpretations of "need" give rise to substantially different rationing principles. The most common practice is to define need in terms of the severity of the clinical illness, such as life-threatening illness, i.e. prolonging life is more urgent than enhancing life [2].

A more expansive definition of "need" as ill health includes both immediate pain and suffering (i.e. bad hip) and an imminent threat to life such as a heart attack. In this context, need is understood as an individual's immediate level of ill health [3].

These two rules are often called the "Rules of Rescue." Rescuing all individuals in need may not always be possible, and saving one person may entail the consequence that others cannot be rescued. When examining need principles, it is crucial to underscore that numerous rationing decisions demand both a comparative assessment of the relative level of need and a binary judgment regarding the presence or absence of a need. A third option involves expanding the interpretation of need as ill health even further by adopting a more extensive time perspective. This might involve considering an individual's entire lifetime of ill health rather than focusing solely on their immediate situation, such as ill health in the next year or so.

Need as Capacity to Benefit

Economists argue that any definition of need solely based on ill health is inadequate, as it overlooks the consideration of the potential benefit that healthcare might bring. Some economists propose two alternative definitions of the need to address this issue.

The first proposal suggests reinterpreting need directly in terms of an individual's capacity to gain health from treatment. This interpretation would involve ranking patients according to health gain, aligning with a maximising principle (disregarding indirect health consequences). A (proportionate) need principle ensures healthcare is allocated to those with lesser needs.

A practical approach might involve a lottery where the probability of treatment is proportional to the capacity to benefit, maintaining proportionality in expected healthcare distribution.

Critics argue that identifying needs with a capacity to benefit could result in bias against those requiring expensive treatments. If two individuals, A and B, have equal needs (capacity to benefit), but treating A is more expensive than B, distributing expenditure based on capacity to benefit might prioritise B over A. To address this, it is proposed that need should be interpreted as the cost of treating the patient to exhaust the capacity to benefit [4, 5].

Maximising the Benefit Principle

In accordance with maximising principles, justice dictates that healthcare distribution should aim to achieve the most favourable outcomes, although various maximising principles evaluate consequences differently. Economists favour maximising principles as they align with a broadly utilitarian approach, albeit distinct from classical utilitarianism, and align well with the consequentialist logic inherent in the classical model of rational choice that underlies standard economic theory. The implications of these principles always hinge on estimates made regarding the likely consequences of different courses of action.

One common maximising principle in this context is to optimise aggregate population health. In the rationing exercise, applying this principle would essentially prioritise treating the patient expected to gain the most total health over their remaining lifespan, considering potential indirect consequences for others' health (e.g. resources freed up for treating other patients). The specific implications depend significantly on the estimates made regarding the expected health gain [6].

A more expansive maximising principle is to optimise wellbeing or flourishing, encompassing elements of well-being beyond health. This does not necessarily align with classical utilitarianism, as wellbeing can be interpreted in terms of "objective" capabilities (such as the ability to set and achieve goals, interact with others, etc.) as well as subjective pleasures [7].

Egalitarian Principle

In this principle, healthcare resources should be distributed to diminish health inequalities. Most proponents of egalitarian principles do not advocate equality as the sole objective; instead, they prefer combining the pursuit of equality with other justice principles, such as maximising health. One form of egalitarian principle is the "fair innings" argument, asserting that everyone is entitled to a similarly long and healthy life. A rigid principle of equalising lifetime health, without considering other justice principles. Another type of egalitarian principle concentrates on equalising individuals' opportunities for lifetime health, considering freedom of choice and autonomy in decisions influencing health, rather than focusing solely on attained levels of health.

Another way to think about equality is to focus on equal opportunities for health, acknowledging individuals' choices and autonomy. This way of thinking about equality is different from the way we usually think about it, because it focuses more on what people choose not to do, like leading an unhealthy lifestyle. In this way, justice would be done if those people experienced lower levels of health [8, 9].

Combination

The ethical decision-making process often incorporates a secondary principle when the primary one lacks a definitive answer. Some authors propose a combined principle that merges a specific (life-saving) needs principle with a lottery principle. The primary emphasis is on saving lives by addressing immediate threats to life. Yet, if multiple individuals share an equal immediate threat to life and resources are constrained, the secondary principle of a lottery is invoked. This approach aims to find a middle ground, ensuring a balance between the urgency of addressing immediate life-threatening situations and the fair allocation of resources when confronted with equal needs [10].

A second approach to combining principles involves assigning weights to two principles without one having absolute priority over the other. A quantifiable combination principle of this nature, for reducing inequalities in lifetime health and the maximising principle for aggregate health. The ranking of patients in the rationing exercise would hinge on the relative weights assigned to these principles, indicating society's aversion to inequality. Assuming mild aversion to inequality, the ranking is mainly determined by health maximisation only [8]. Others advocate a combination of the need principle, which involves distributing in proportion to immediate ill health, along with the maximising principle aimed at maximising health [4].

For healthcare services eligible for public funding, the approach involves assessing the relative effectiveness of each service. The services are ranked based on their effectiveness, and the healthcare budget determines the cutoff point. Only services ranked above this threshold receive funding, emphasising a balance between maximising health (by excluding relatively ineffective services) and distributing in proportion to capacity to benefit (by including relatively effective services even if not cost-effective) [3].

Possibly the healthcare system should be structured to bring everyone as close as possible to a decent minimum level of health, termed "normal species functioning in line with Rawls theory of justice. There is an opportunity for additional philosophical exploration in formulating new theories of justice in healthcare rationing that are more diverse than distribution based on need or health maximisation, aligning better with the common moral intuitions of the public [11, 12].

References

1. Cookson R, Dolan P. Public views on health care rationing: a group discussion study. Health Policy. 1999;49:63–74.
2. British Medical Association. Philosophy and practice of medical ethics. London: British Medical Association; 1988.
3. Hadorn D. Setting health care priorities in Oregon: cost-effectiveness meets the rule of rescue. JAMA J Am Med Assoc. 1991;265:2218–25.

4. Broome J. Good, fairness and QALYs. In: Bell M, Mendus S, editors. Philosophy and medical welfare, vol. 23. Cambridge: University of Cambridge Press; 1988. p. 57.
5. Culyer AJ. Need—is a consensus possible? J Med Ethics. 1998;24:77–80.
6. Culyer AJ. The principle objective of the NHS should be to maximise aggregate health. In: New B, editor. Rationing: talk and action in health care. London: King's Fund and British Medical Journal Publishing Group; 1997.
7. Sen A. Capability and Well-being. In: Nussbaum M, Sen A, editors. The quality of life. Oxford: Clarendon Press; 1993.
8. Williams A. Intergenerational equity: an exploration of the 'fair innings' argument. Health Econ. 1997;6(2):117–32.
9. LeGrand J. Equity and choice. London: Harper Collins; 1991.
10. Harris J. The value of life: an introduction to medical ethics. London: Routledge; 1985.
11. Hare R. Health care policy: some options. In: Hare R, editor. Essays on bioethics. Oxford: Clarendon Press; 1993. p. 209–11.
12. Rawls J. A theory of justice. Cambridge, Mass: Harvard University Press; 1971.

Chapter 12
Understanding Medical Epistemology

The word "epistemology" etymologically comes from two Greek words: epistēmē (knowledge) and logos (study) and is conventionally defined as "Theory of Knowledge." Was first introduced by James F. Ferrier (1808–1864), English philosopher and based on thoughts of Georg Berkeley introduced the term epistemology, begins the development of his thought with the axiom: "Along with whatever any intelligence knows, it must, as the ground or condition of its knowledge, have some cognisance of itself." And will conclude by stating: "All absolute existences are contingent except one; in other words, there is One, but only one, Absolute Existence, which is strictly necessary; and that existence is a supreme and infinite and everlasting Mind in synthesis with all things" [1].

Medicine has evolved throughout history, adapting to changes in society, advancements in science, and technological innovations.

Medical epistemology, a subset of epistemology, deals with the nature, scope, and limits of knowledge in the field of medicine. It explores how medical knowledge is acquired, justified, and applied.

Although ancient agrarian societies in Mesopotamia and Egypt did not prioritise the acquisition of knowledge through empirical evidence, they inadvertently generated such knowledge. It was only when Ancient Greek natural philosophers like Thales of Miletus (ca. 624–546 BC) emerged that a strictly theoretical and scientific approach to understanding nature was introduced. There are, and have been, many myths about science and scientists. One version of the myth of the lonely genius. It regards the brilliant scientist as a man who, in a moment of inspiration, unconditioned by his social setting, creates a new idea that once and for all solves a scientific problem. Another version of the myth disregards the surrounding milieu but stresses a supposedly calm and disinterested use of a rational faculty. Despite the existence of scientific geniuses, these views heavily underrate the role played by technological, economic, political, social, and cultural circumstances in the development of science. Even though some famous scientists have in fact had the experience of receiving a revolutionary idea like a flash of lightning, it should be remembered that even real light flashes have their very determinate existential

S. Abbas, *Medical Ethics*, https://doi.org/10.1007/978-981-96-9199-9_12

preconditions. Louis Pasteur is often quoted as saying: "In the field of observation, chance favours only the prepared mind." This is a variation of the more general theme that luck is the reward of the prepared mind. To invent or discover something new, people must be in a state of readiness [2].

Knowledge can be sourced from various avenues, including:

Facts and Figures: This involves utilising measurements, numerical data, and statistics, often found in evidence-based research.

Observation and Empirical Thought: Knowledge can be gained by recognising patterns and making direct measurements using one's own senses. The scientific method heavily relies on this approach.

Experience: Past personal experiences, even if anecdotal, shape what we consider to be true. While not always valued in evidence-based medicine, anecdotal evidence can be influential.

Hands-On Learning (Heuristics): Knowledge can be acquired through practical, hands-on experience. For example, knowing how to perform a medical procedure based on previous learning.

Learning from Others: Gathering information from various sources, including experts, books, education, media, and advertising. Social connections and affiliations also contribute to our understanding of truth, as does cultural and traditional knowledge.

Narratives and Art: Stories and artistic expressions are powerful tools for conveying knowledge and have been used throughout history to inform future generations.

Instinct and Personality: Sometimes, individuals simply know something based on their instincts or personal characteristics.

Intuition and Inspiration: In the realm of conventional medicine, intuition and inspiration can play a role in diagnosis and treatment decisions.

Serendipity, Chance, Luck: Occasionally, important discoveries or knowledge emerge from unexpected or chance occurrences.

Collective Consciousness: Some believe that knowledge can spread across a group when one member develops it, contributing to collective understanding.

Contemplation and Reflection: Mindful awareness and intentional reflection, using various methods or traditions, can enhance one's understanding of different subjects.

Spiritual and Personal Means: Personal beliefs and spirituality can also be a significant source of knowledge, often on deeply personal matters. These diverse sources of knowledge highlight the complexity of how individuals come to understand and perceive truth in various aspects of life, including healthcare [2, 3].

Here are some key aspects to elaborate on:

Sources of Medical Knowledge Medical knowledge is obtained from various sources, including clinical experience, scientific research, patient testimonies, and medical literature. Medical epistemology examines the reliability and credibility of these sources. It also investigates how medical knowledge is transmitted from one generation of healthcare practitioners to the next.

Evidence-Based Medicine A significant focus of medical epistemology is evidence-based medicine (EBM). EBM emphasises the use of the best available evidence from systematic research, clinical trials, and patient data to inform medical decision-making. Philosophers and practitioners of medicine explore questions related to the quality of evidence, the hierarchy of evidence, and the ethical implications of EBM.

Uncertainty and Probability Medicine often deals with uncertainty. Medical epistemology delves into how healthcare professionals manage uncertainty when making diagnoses and treatment decisions. It also examines the role of probability and statistics in medical reasoning, especially in predicting outcomes and assessing risks.

Clinical Reasoning and Expertise The process of clinical reasoning, where healthcare professionals gather and interpret clinical data to make diagnoses and treatment plans, is a central concern of medical epistemology. It explores the development of medical expertise, heuristics, and biases in clinical decision-making.

Medical Ethics and Epistemology: Medical epistemology intersects with medical ethics in various ways. Ethical questions arise when considering the limits of medical knowledge, the communication of uncertain or probabilistic information to patients, and the ethics of conducting medical research. Philosophers in this field explore the responsibilities of healthcare professionals in light of epistemic uncertainty.

Clinical Guidelines and Protocols The development and use of clinical guidelines and protocols play a role in standardising medical practice. Medical epistemology assesses the epistemic basis for these guidelines, including how they are derived from evidence and expert consensus. It also examines the role of clinical guidelines in balancing individualised patient care with population-level health outcomes.

Patient-Centred Care An evolving area of interest is patient-centred care, which emphasises the importance of involving patients in medical decision-making. Medical epistemology explores the epistemic dimension of shared decision-making, informed consent, and the integration of patients' values and preferences into clinical practice.

Cross-Disciplinary Inquiry Given the complex nature of medicine, medical epistemology often engages with other disciplines, such as philosophy of science, philosophy of biology, sociology of medicine, and cognitive science. These interdisciplinary approaches help address the unique epistemic challenges in medicine.

Medical epistemology is a branch of philosophy that critically examines how medical knowledge is generated, validated, and applied. It grapples with the inherent uncertainty in medicine and seeks to improve the quality of medical decision-making while addressing ethical concerns related to knowledge and practice in healthcare.

We'll distinguish between (1) how science develops and (2) how it evolves.

1. Does science always accumulate by adding one bit of knowledge to another, or are there sometimes discontinuities and great leaps? The history of science seems to show that in one respect scientific communities (with the theories and kind of research they are bearers of) behave very much like political communities (with the ideologies and kind of economic-political structures they are bearers of). Mostly, there is an evolutionary process, but now and then there are revolutions. In some cases, historians talk of half a century-long extended revolutions such as the first industrial revolution around the turn of the eighteenth century and the scientific revolution in the middle the seventeenth century. In other cases, such as the French revolution of 1789 and the Russian one of 1917, the revolutions are extremely rapid. In science, most revolutions are of the slow kind; one case of a rapid revolution is Einstein's relativistic revolution in physics.
2. When those who search for causes behind scientific development think they can find an overarching one-factor theory, they quarrel about whether the causes are factors such as technological, economic, political, social, and cultural conditions external to the scientific community (externalism) or factors such as the social milieu and the ideas and/or methodologies within a scientific community (internalism).

Medicine is not perceived as an independent science but rather as a body of knowledge, methods, and competencies drawn from various fields, encompassing the humanities and social sciences. Its aim is to study and address the health-disease continuum in a holistic manner, recognising that this process extends beyond the boundaries of the biological and social realms. While its underlying factors are rooted in the social context, they encompass biological and even spiritual aspects. Consequently, medicine emerges as a social practice where art, science, and technique come together to safeguard or renew an individual's state of well-being.

The context in which medical science knowledge evolves undergoes an epistemological transformation, becoming a multifaceted, ever-changing realm. This transformation arises from the integration of the art, science, and technical dimensions within the realm of medical practice as a whole. Consequently, this holistic fusion of the art-science-technical aspects exemplifies the progress of scientific understanding within the realm of medicine and health sciences. It is through professional practice that this intricate interplay of elements becomes apparent, representing a reality where two fundamental factors come to the forefront: the evolution of techniques and the imperative to comprehend the environment in which the health-disease process unfolds.

The process of constructing rational explanations for reality through the subject-object-subject relationship is not confined solely to philosophy or abstract theories of knowledge; it also finds relevance in various scientific disciplines. An example of this can be found in medicine, where the understanding of diseases has evolved over time within different cultural contexts. Each civilisation had to interpret and address diseases based on their beliefs, knowledge, and intellectual frameworks, which sometimes diverged significantly from established scientific norms.

The subject-object-subject dynamic, which underpins the exploration of medical sciences, mitigates the traditional dichotomy between natural sciences and social sciences. Instead, it leads to diverse methodological strategies for grasping the health-disease process, from quantitative to qualitative analyses and from explanation to comprehension [3, 4].

To understand reality, it is important to establish a logical framework of knowledge. This framework not only aids in recognising the limits of scientific knowledge in the health sciences but also encourages us to explore thought-provoking questions.

Epistemologists investigate the origins and organisational principles of sciences from logical, historical, and sociological perspectives. They analyse explanations rooted in belief systems and testimonies, which hinge on concepts such as causality, certainty, coherence, fallibility, illusion, inference, intellectual virtue, introspection, intuition, sense, memory, reasoning, relativity, reality, and truth. In this context, a study was conducted to identify the foundational epistemology components of medicine [4, 5].

While various perspectives on matters of knowledge had been discussed in Greek philosophy, it was not until the modern era that the theory of knowledge emerged as an independent discipline. Philosophers like John Locke, George Berkeley, and David Hume, embarked on systematic inquiries into human knowledge, addressing five core issues: the feasibility of knowledge, the sources of knowledge, the nature of knowledge, the different modes of knowledge, and the criteria for determining truth. It was not until the year 1781, with the publication of Immanuel Kant's "Critique of Pure Reason," that the critical underpinnings of scientific knowledge in the realm of nature were elucidated.

The development of the theory of knowledge, or epistemology, can be traced back to ancient Greek philosophy, where various perspectives on knowledge were explored. However, it was not until the modern era that epistemology took shape as an independent and systematic discipline. This transformation can be attributed to the works of influential philosophers such as John Locke, George Berkeley, and David Hume.

These philosophers engaged in rigorous investigations into the nature of human knowledge, tackling five fundamental questions that continue to shape contemporary epistemological inquiries:

Feasibility of Knowledge: They examined whether knowledge acquisition was possible and under what conditions. This involved delving into the limitations and boundaries of what humans can know.

Sources of Knowledge: They explored the origins of knowledge, considering whether it arises from sensory experiences, innate ideas, or other sources. This investigation aimed to uncover the foundational elements upon which knowledge is built.

Nature of Knowledge: Philosophers questioned what knowledge actually consists of. This included inquiries into the structure and composition of knowledge, distinguishing it from belief or mere opinion.

Modes of Knowledge: They investigated the different ways in which knowledge can be acquired and categorised. This encompassed areas such as empirical knowledge gained through observation and a priori knowledge deduced through reason alone.

Criteria for Determining Truth: Philosophers sought to establish the criteria or standards by which the truth of a belief or claim could be determined. This involved scrutinising the reliability of evidence and the conditions under which something could be considered true.

Despite the significant progress made by Locke, Berkeley, and Hume in addressing these questions, it was Immanuel Kant's groundbreaking work, "Critique of Pure Reason," published in 1781, that marked a turning point in the field of epistemology. Kant's critique provided a critical and systematic examination of the foundations of scientific knowledge, particularly in the domain of the natural sciences. He introduced the concept of a priori knowledge and emphasised the role of human cognition and perception in shaping our understanding of reality.

Kant's work laid the groundwork for future developments in epistemology and continues to influence contemporary discussions on the nature, limits, and justification of knowledge. His ideas also extended beyond epistemology, impacting various other fields of philosophy, including metaphysics and ethics, making him one of the most significant figures in the history of philosophy [5–8].

To know something, you must understand it connects with the broader theory of knowledge. This theory explores the analytical problem of knowledge, which examines the prerequisites that are both essential and adequate for affirming that an individual possesses particular knowledge. We rely on the epistemological examination rooted in the classical theory of knowledge. According to this classical theory of knowledge, a statement qualifies as knowledge only when it fulfils two indispensable criteria: justification and truth. In other words, a belief embedded within a statement must be not only justified but also true for that statement to be considered a manifestation of knowledge. This epistemological perspective is instrumental in establishing the conditions that delineate when a belief can be classified as knowledge and when a statement can be deemed rational [9, 10].

Epistemology, in its evolving relationship with other branches of philosophy, sociology of science, and history of science, has seen enrichment in its domain of inquiry. Mario Bunge introduced the concept of "new epistemology," defining it as a philosophical branch concerned with the study of scientific research and its output, scientific knowledge. This new perspective has given rise to various branches, each addressing distinct philosophical aspects of epistemology.

Moreover, these branches not only engage with issues pertaining to scientific knowledge but also delve into the epistemological challenges posed by different scientific disciplines, leading to the emergence of regional epistemologies, epistemology has also been shaped as a reflection on science itself [11].

Epistemology addresses the constitution of valid scientific knowledge and explores the relationships between the subject and the object in understanding reality, i.e. epistemology seeks to uncover how knowledge connects with the real world.

In this pursuit of knowledge, Mario Bunge outlines the Ontological Principles of Science:

1. There exists a world external to the knowing subject.
2. The world comprises material objects.
3. Properties are attributed to specific entities; there are no inherent properties.
4. Objects form associations and systems.
5. Systems interact with others in certain ways and remain isolated from others.
6. Everything, including systems, undergoes change.
7. Nothing emerges from nothing, and nothing is entirely reduced to nothingness.
8. All phenomena adhere to objective laws.
9. Various types of laws exist, such as causal and probabilistic, operating within the same level or across different levels.
10. Multiple levels of organisation exist, spanning the physical, chemical, biological, social, technical, etc.

Epistemological Principles of Science:

1. Reality is partially knowable.
2. Scientific research can expand our knowledge of reality.
3. Different sources or modes of knowledge exist, including sensory experience, intuition, action, and reason.
4. Scientific theories serve as representations (symbolic, more or less true) of presumed real entities.
5. The truthfulness of scientific theories is provisionally determined through observations and experiments [12].

With the emergence of modern science, a clear differentiation was established among various forms of knowledge, including everyday knowledge (empirical truths), philosophical knowledge (rational truths), religious knowledge (faith-based truths), and scientific knowledge, which is grounded in empirical truths derived from sensory experience and rational truths through necessary demonstrations. In this context, the scientific method gained importance as a means to distinguish scientific knowledge from other forms of knowledge. This method involved verifying hypotheses through techniques such as induction, the hypothetical-deductive approach, and experimental procedures [13].

It is essential to understand the importance of understanding and respecting these different perspectives to develop effective decision strategies that both clinicians and patients can agree on. It highlights various ways of knowing, including facts and figures, observation, personal experience, learning from others, and more.

Epistemological clashes, where different perspectives collide, are common in healthcare, especially regarding diagnoses, treatments, and healthcare decisions. To address these clashes, the text suggests:

1. Understanding the patient's perspective by asking questions and reflecting on their beliefs.
2. Being clear about your own beliefs and opinions without being judgmental.
3. Ensuring patient safety and considering the potential harm of preferred treatments.
4. Sharing evidence-based information and recommending reliable resources.
5. Admitting when you don't know and being mindful of your emotions during interactions.

Ultimately, patient-centred care involves acknowledging diverse perspectives and building strong therapeutic relationships to improve patient outcomes.

References

1. Ferrier JF. Institutes of methaphysics. The theory of knowing and being. Edinburgh: William Blackwood and Sons; 1854.
2. https://ki.se/sites/default/files/2019/12/01_Johanson-Medicine.pdf.
3. Sendrail M. Historia cultural de la enfermedad. España: Editorial Espasa-Calpe; 1983.
4. Malinowski B. Magia, ciencia y religión. México: Editorial Planeta-De Agostini; 1985.
5. Locke J. Ensayo sobre el entendimiento humano. 2nd ed. México, D.F.: Fondo de Cultura Económica; 2005.
6. Berkeley G. Tratado sobre los principios del conocimiento humano. Madrid: Alianza Editorial; 1992.
7. Hume D. An enquiry concerning human understanding. New York: Oxford University Press; 1999.
8. Kant I. Critique of pure reason. London: Penguin Group; 2007.
9. Gettier EL. Is justified true belief knowledge? Analysis. 1963;23:121–3.
10. Nozick R. Philosophical explanations. Cambridge, USA: Harvard University Press; 1983.
11. Laudan L. Beyond positivism and relativism: theory, method and evidence. Westview Press; 1996.
12. Bunge M. Epistemología. México: Siglo XXI Editores; 1997.
13. Kuhn TS. The structure of scientific revolutions. 4th ed. Chicago: The University of Chicago Press; 2012.

Chapter 13
Law and Medicine: Aristotle, Kant, JS Mill, and Rawls

The relationship between classical philosophy and modern medical ethics is intricate.

What are the philosophical foundations of medical ethics? The term ethics is derived from Greek. It means "character" or "disposition." It is used in Aristotle to denote those aspects of one's character that, through appropriate moral training, develop into virtue. What are the philosophical foundations of medical ethics? The term ethics is derived from Greek. The noun meaning "character" or "disposition." It is used in Aristotle to denote those aspects of one's character that, through appropriate moral training, develop into virtues. Is related to the adjective denoting someone or something that relates to disposition, e.g., a philosophical study on character. Ethics is concerned with what is good for individuals and society. It involves developing, systematising, defending, and recommending concepts of right and wrong behaviour.

Prominent philosophers like Aristotle, Kant, Mill, and Rawls have significantly influenced modern medical ethics.

1. Virtue Ethics: Emphasises cultivating virtues like compassion in healthcare. Kant:
2. Deontological Ethics: Focuses on duty and treating patients with respect. Mill:
3. Utilitarianism: Considers overall well-being in healthcare decisions. Rawls:
4. Justice as Fairness: Prioritises fairness and equality in healthcare policies.

Modern medical ethics applies these philosophies in areas like informed consent, end-of-life care, resource allocation, healthcare equity, and nurturing virtues in healthcare.

In examining Western ethical theories, we need to elaborate on three distinct philosophical approaches: Aristotle's virtue ethics, Kant's duty-based ethics, and utilitarianism. Each of these philosophical perspectives offers unique insights into moral decision-making and ethical conduct [1].

Aristotle's Virtue Ethics: Aristotle's ethical framework aims at human happiness (eudaimonia) as the ultimate goal, emphasising fulfilling and purposeful activity. To

S. Abbas, *Medical Ethics*, https://doi.org/10.1007/978-981-96-9199-9_13

achieve happiness, individuals must align their actions with their rational human function, maintaining a balance between reason and emotion. Virtues, such as courage and honesty, are central, representing the mean between extremes and developed through habituation and practice.

Kant's Duty-Based Ethics: Kant's ethics revolves around duty and universal moral principles. The categorical imperative dictates that individuals should act according to maxims that could be universal laws without contradiction. Kant's deontological approach prioritises moral duty over consequences, emphasising patient autonomy and the duty to respect human dignity in medical ethics.

Utilitarianism: Utilitarianism seeks to maximise overall happiness or utility, focusing on the greatest good for the greatest number [1–4].

John Stuart Mill introduced the concept of higher and lower pleasures, considering both quantity and quality of happiness. Utilitarianism informs decisions in healthcare resource allocation and ethical dilemmas.

In summary, these ethical theories—Aristotle's virtue ethics, Kant's duty-based ethics, and utilitarianism—offer distinct perspectives for analysing and addressing moral issues in medical ethics, spanning character development, universal duties, and consequences. Understanding these frameworks is essential for navigating complex healthcare ethical dilemmas and aligning medical decisions with ethical value.

Aristotle's Virtue Ethics: Aristotle's ethics centres on happiness (eudaimonia) as the ultimate goal.

Kant's ethical perspective is firmly deontological, placing duty at the core of morality. He establishes a profound connection between freedom and ethics, asserting that our capacity for reason and autonomy defines our freedom. This capacity allows us to establish our moral principles, rendering us morally accountable. Kant asserts that our moral agency arises from our faculties of reason and autonomy, underscoring the uniqueness and irreplaceability of each individual. Consequently, Kant staunchly upholds individual rights [1].

Additionally, Kant highlights our ability to establish the moral law, a process through which we determine our duties as moral agents. Kantian ethics remains indifferent to consequences; it revolves around fulfilling our obligations. This ethical framework relies on what Kant terms the categorical imperative, the supreme moral principle.

Kant's Categorical Imperative

Kant's moral theory encompasses two formulations of the categorical imperative. When confronted with moral dilemmas, individuals must evaluate whether their actions align with these formulations. The first formulation dictates that our actions should be such that the principles (maxims) behind them could be universal laws. If a maxim cannot be applied universally, the action is morally impermissible. For example, when contemplating theft, one must assess whether a world where everyone steals is acceptable; it is not, as it undermines the concept of private property. This test ensures logical consistency and fairness in maxims.

The second formulation underscores the importance of treating all individuals, including oneself, as ends in themselves, never as mere means. It mandates respecting human dignity, assisting others in achieving their goals when possible, and refraining from exploiting them for personal gain. Kant emphasizes the significance of honoring human autonomy and rationality. His two formulations underscore critical aspects of his moral theory, including fairness, justice, individual rights, and consistency.

Strengths of Kant's Approach

Provides an explanation for the inherent wrongness of actions like slavery and rape.

Offers clarity regarding objections to paternalistic laws or behaviours.

Supports the concept of universal human rights.

Emphasises human moral responsibility.

Challenges with Kant's Approach

Questions arise regarding whether it consistently prioritises justice above all else.

Complexity surrounds the concept of autonomy and its applicability.

Some critics argue that it disregards the importance of consequences entirely.

Kant's approach limits the moral community to those who are autonomous and rational [4–6].

Kant's ethical perspective is firmly deontological, placing duty at the core of morality. He establishes a profound connection between freedom and ethics, asserting that our capacity for reason and autonomy defines our freedom. This capacity allows us to establish our moral principles, rendering us morally accountable. Kant asserts that our moral agency arises from our faculties of reason and autonomy, underscoring the uniqueness and irreplaceability of each individual. Consequently, Kant staunchly upholds individual rights [4].

Additionally, Kant highlights our ability to establish the moral law, a process through which we determine our duties as moral agents. Kantian ethics remains indifferent to consequences; it revolves around fulfilling our obligations. This ethical framework relies on what Kant terms the categorical imperative, the supreme moral principle.

References

1. Jonsen AR. A short history of medical ethics. 2000.
2. Mill JS. Utilitarianism, liberty, and representative government. 1948.
3. Rawls J. Rational and full autonomy. J Philos. 1980;77:515.
4. Kant E. Foundations of the metaphysics of morals and what is enlightenment? 1959.
5. Altman MC. Kant and applied ethics: the uses and limits of Kant's practical philosophy. 2014.
6. Beauchamp TL, et al. Principles of biomedical ethics. 2013.

Chapter 14
Patient's Rights

The Principles

The origins of ethical principles, especially those concerning physicians, trace back to ancient civilisations like Mesopotamia, Egypt, and Greece. Ethical discussions within these cultures date back to around 2340 BCE with the writings of individuals like Nefer-seshem-re and flourished during Greece's golden age in the fifth century BCE.

Similarly, considerations of physicians' ethical responsibilities have ancient roots, with examples like the tomb inscription of Nenkh-Sekhmet around 2400 BCE and the Hippocratic school's writings in the fifth century BCE. Deontological ethics, which emphasise duty and obligation and have a significant influence on modern law and healthcare, emerged later with Immanuel Kant's works in the late eighteenth century.

On the other hand, human rights writings developed relatively later in history. Political rights for Western citizens were first established by the Magna Carta in 1215 CE. Enlightenment thinkers such as John Locke in the 1600s and 1700s introduced human rights into Western scholarly and philosophical discourse. Patient rights, although earlier established through civil suits after adverse healthcare outcomes in 1374 CE, were formally recognised by the First Geneva Convention in 1864, primarily for wounded soldiers. The World Health Organization, founded in 1948, created the first comprehensive bill of health rights, applicable to all individuals, marking a significant step in the expansion of patient rights. Patient rights find their basis in these preexisting ethical principles [1].

In modern Western medicine, core ethical principles include:

1. Beneficence: This principle involves acting in the best interest of the patient during diagnosis and treatment. It encompasses both physical and holistic care, addressing emotional, social, and spiritual well-being. However, conflicts may arise between a physician's intent for beneficence and patient autonomy,

S. Abbas, *Medical Ethics*, https://doi.org/10.1007/978-981-96-9199-9_14

necessitating clear communication and informed decision-making when disagreements occur.

2. Autonomy (literally "self-rule") refers to the capacity to live according to one's own reasons and motives. Concerning the autonomy of ordinary citizens, Western society has undergone a radical change in the last 350 years. Before the Enlightenment, most persons lived under the rule of a monarch or similar type of authority. Early Enlightenment philosophers (e.g., Hobbes, Locke, and Rousseau) advocated what is now called social contract theory. This is the view that persons' moral and political obligations should depend on an agreement amongst themselves regarding which rules will hold in their particular society. Later philosophers argued for individual autonomy to an even greater degree than championed by social contract theorists. Autonomy as a fundamental aspect of human existence was advanced largely by two moral and social philosophers, John Stuart Mill (early nineteenth century; of the school of utilitarian liberalism) and Immanuel Kant, respectively. Kant proposed that each person of sound mind should first live in moral autonomy, imposing moral decisions regarding himself or herself on himself or herself and secondly allow all other persons to do the same. Mill advocated autonomy with regard to a person's capacity to govern oneself, and subsequent philosophers and jurists expanded autonomy to include other forms of self-expression. Western post-Enlightenment philosophy and law are no longer concerned with whether autonomy in its various forms is a human right but instead to whom it extends and to what degree. A patient who can defend his or her judgments has the right to make decisions that do not coincide with what the physician believes is beneficial to that patient. This philosophical concept has become a legal right essentially throughout the Western world. As legal precedents have advanced the requirements for patient autonomy to a greater degree than the requirements for healthcare provider beneficence, patient autonomy has arguably become the dominant principle affecting patient rights. For example, a patient may refuse treatment that the physician deems to be an act of beneficence. In such cases, the unwritten social contract between patient and physician requires that medical professionals still attempt to inform the patient of the potential consequences of proceeding against medical advice. A patient's autonomy is violated when family members or members of a healthcare team pressure a patient or when they act on the patient's behalf without the patient's permission (in a non-emergency situation).
3. Complementary to beneficence, nonmaleficence seeks to ensure a patient will be no worse off (physically, emotionally, or otherwise) after treatment than before. Nonmaleficence dates to the medical writings of the early Egyptians, as cited earlier. The Hippocratic Oath lists specific acts of nonmaleficence, including euthanasia, abortion, an attempt by the professional at procedures outside of his area of expertise, stealing property, making sexual advances, and violating privacy. The consideration of whether a treatment plan is or is not malevolent extends to all types of treatments, including medications, physical manipulations, and invasive procedures. In relation to other ethical principles, nonmaleficence most commonly conflicts with beneficence. Despite the potential reason

why treatment is beneficial, the therapy may have unintended harm. Examples include procedures in which a surgeon must cut into a patient's body or certain drugs (such as chemotherapies). The body is essentially poisoned so that it may have the opportunity to heal later. In each case, the odds and degree of harm must be weighed against that of benefit. Physicians cannot control all responses to treatments. So a physician can still act under the principle of non-maleficence if the physician takes measures to minimise the chances of harm and informs the patient prior to taking the risk so that the patient has the opportunity to accept or decline the risk.

4. Justice in healthcare, specifically "distributive justice," ensures fair and equal treatment for all patients. It mandates that individuals' rights be respected and that all patients in a given situation are treated impartially, regardless of their identity. Healthcare laws and policies rely on this principle to ensure universal access to life-preserving care, including emergency situations. Some authorities have expanded the scope of healthcare justice beyond emergencies. Distributive justice, as defined by John Rawls, embodies equal respect for individuals, ensuring that those with similar needs receive the same rights and services, while those with greater needs receive more substantial benefits [3].

The Basics

Private institutions often create their own patient declarations or bills of rights. These documents serve to educate patients about their rights and may include additional rights beyond those mandated by law. While the term "bill" typically refers to a document evaluated for becoming a law, it can informally refer to any list of declared rights.

For instance, Indiana University Health has its own patient bill of rights, which outlines various patient rights. The health and well-being of patients rely on a collaborative partnership between patients and physicians, characterised by mutual respect. Patients play a vital role in this alliance by fulfilling certain responsibilities, such as seeking medical care and being open and honest with their physicians [2].

In turn, physicians can best contribute to this respectful partnership by acting as advocates for their patients and honouring patients' rights. These rights encompass:

1. The right to be treated with courtesy, respect, and dignity, receiving timely and responsive attention to their needs.
2. The right to receive comprehensive information from their physicians and the opportunity to discuss the advantages, disadvantages, and costs of appropriate treatment options, including the potential consequences of choosing not to undergo treatment. Patients should expect guidance from their physicians based on objective professional judgment.
3. The right to ask questions about their health status or recommended treatments when they have uncertainties and to receive clear answers.

4. The right to make decisions regarding their healthcare, and to have these choices respected. Patients with decision-making capacity have the autonomy to accept or decline recommended medical interventions.
5. The right to privacy and confidentiality, with the physician and staff respecting their personal information.
6. The right to access copies or summaries of their medical records.
7. The right to seek a second opinion.
8. The right to be informed of any potential conflicts of interest that their physician may have in relation to their care.
9. The right to continuity of care. Patients should anticipate that their physician will collaborate in coordinating necessary medical care with other healthcare professionals, and that the physician will provide sufficient notice and assistance in arranging alternative care if they decide to discontinue treatment when it is still medically necessary.

The patient–provider relationship is built on trust, with the patient relying on the healthcare professional to act in their best interests due to the professional's expertise. This relationship is inherently imbalanced in power, as the patient often knows little about vital medical matters. Patients vary in their preference for involvement in this relationship. Four models of patient-physician relationships exist:

1. Paternalistic: The doctor decides on the patient's behalf, with minimal patient involvement.
2. Interpretive: The doctor understands the patient's goals and values, offering options that align with them, while the patient remains passive.
3. Informative: The doctor provides information to aid the patient's decision-making, leaving the final choice to the patient.
4. Deliberative: In this collaborative model, the doctor and patient work together as equals to achieve healthcare goals and uphold values, offering the most patient-centric approach [2, 3].

Patient rights in modern medicine have evolved through various legal actions. In 1973, the American Hospital Association introduced the first patient bill of rights. While these bills are a step toward protecting patients, they have limited enforceability.

North American countries, including Canada, the United States, and Mexico, have introduced laws to safeguard patient rights, but none has established a comprehensive patient bill of rights, unlike many European nations. Instead, patient rights in North America are often covered under broader human rights legislation, rather than being specific to healthcare.

In 2001, there were unsuccessful attempts in the USA and Canada to pass a dedicated patient bill of rights legislation. Consequently, many states and provinces have developed their own patient rights policies, leading to variations in standards between regions and hospitals. Examples of patient rights are influenced by various ethical principles and can vary depending on the specific context [2].

Informed Consent

Informed consent comprises two key elements: the right to be informed about potential harm to one's body by a hired agent and the right to autonomy. The concept of informing patients about their health status began to gain traction in the nineteenth century. Landmark legal decisions in the twentieth century, such as Canterbury v. Spence, Cobb v. Grant, and Wilkinson v. Vesey, led to the American Medical Association recognising informed consent as a fundamental social policy in 1981, prioritising patient autonomy over healthcare provider beneficence.

Informed consent's origins can be traced back to social contract theorists of the 1600s and 1700s, who argued that patients own their bodies and have the right to decide the risks and costs associated with medical treatments. The traditional medical assumption that physicians know best has shifted to an autonomy-based philosophy, where patients are empowered to make decisions about their care whenever they have the capacity to do so. US courts have even ruled that risks as low as 1% must be disclosed to patients, especially when such risks involve life-altering complications or death.

In the United States, both federal and state legislation protect the right to informed consent. However, state laws often provide more detailed specifications regarding informed consent rights. Enforcement of these rights often occurs through tort claims brought by patients against healthcare providers in the judicial branch.

Documentation of informed consent discussions typically includes five key elements: the nature of the procedure, risks and benefits, reasonable alternatives, risks and benefits of alternatives, and an assessment of the patient's understanding of these elements [4].

Emergency Medical Care

Emergency medical care is a fundamental right grounded in the principles of beneficence and justice, with its origins dating back to the Hippocratic Writings. Regardless of a patient's ability to pay, life-saving measures must be administered until the patient is stabilised. However, the application of this right can vary among medical institutions.

Institutions may differ in their definitions of what constitutes an emergency and when a patient can be considered stable enough to discontinue immediate treatment or require assurance of future compensation for further care. Consequently, patient experiences may vary from one institution to another. In the United States, the right to receive emergency medical treatment was established in 1986 as part of the Consolidated Omnibus Budget Reconciliation Act (COBRA).

Both patients and physicians have the right to refuse treatment for different reasons. A patient may decline treatment that the healthcare provider believes would be beneficial, asserting their autonomy.

Conversely, a physician may opt not to administer a treatment due to concerns about causing more harm than good, aligned with the principle of non-maleficence. Physician refusal depends on the specific situation and is primarily addressed at the state level through statutes or legal decisions.

In both cases, when possible (in non-emergencies), medical professionals must ensure that informed consent is provided regarding the treatment refusal [5].

Confidentiality in healthcare, driven by the physician–patient relationship and respect for autonomy, is a vital aspect of patient care. It ensures that patients can trust their physicians not to disclose sensitive information that could be exploited or harm them in any way, granting patients control over who knows about their health status.

Exceptions to confidentiality arise in cases of imminent danger to the patient or others, as well as certain infectious diseases, such as reportable sexually transmitted infections (STIs) like Human papillomavirus, genital herpes, Chlamydia, gonorrhea, HIV/AIDS, and syphilis. While parental consent is typically required, exceptions apply to contraception, STI treatment, and mental health care [4, 6].

Continuity of Care

Continuity of care empowers patients to make choices about their healthcare providers and treatment plans, fostering patient autonomy and strengthening the patient–physician relationship. It also includes guidance on maintaining health beyond clinical settings and understanding the need for transfers to other facilities or providers when necessary. While not a legal right in the United States, the Affordable Care Act incentivises organisations to promote continuity of care.

Ability to Address Unfair Treatment

Patients and their representatives have the right to voice concerns and seek resolution when healthcare providers fail to address their needs adequately. This right, protected by law in the United States, safeguards patients from treatment prioritising provider interests over patient well-being [4, 6].

In 2010, the US Congress passed the Patient Protection and Affordable Care Act (ACA), with some of its provisions taking effect in subsequent years. Patient rights under the ACA are outlined in various sections of the Code of Federal Regulations.

The ACA introduced several patient rights, including:

1. Access to insurance coverage regardless of preexisting health conditions, often without extra charges, especially for children.
2. Access to many preventive care services at no cost.
3. Access to essential health benefits with no lifetime or annual limits on coverage.

4. The ability to maintain health insurance coverage even when facing illness.
5. Some degree of choice in selecting healthcare providers.
6. Protections against employer retaliation in certain situations.
7. Access to previously uncovered health benefits, including those related to mental health conditions [2, 6, 7].

Patients who leave against medical advice:

1. Assess the patient's decision-making capacity. Ensure they comprehend the information, understand the consequences, and are aware of the risks and benefits associated with their choices, making sure they can communicate this understanding to you.
2. Refrain from blaming or chastising the patient or others for their wish to leave.
3. Offer apologies if the patient has experienced prolonged wait times or delays in their care. Apologising is a simple gesture, while legal actions can be financially costly.
4. Avoid merely instructing the nurse to have the patient sign a generic form and depart. This approach offers limited protection for the healthcare provider.
5. Involve the patient's family and friends in your efforts to persuade the patient to stay.
6. Refrain from expressing frustration or anger to the patient. Instead, sincerely emphasise that your primary concern is their well-being. Assure them that you are supporting their health interests in the face of potential health risks.
7. Document the patient's "informed refusal" of critical diagnostic tests (blood work or scans), procedures (lumbar puncture for ruling out conditions like meningitis or subarachnoid haemorrhage), or treatments (medications or transfusions).
8. Avoid denying treatment, as it may be seen as patient abandonment. Offer the treatment, prescriptions, follow-up appointments, and clear discharge instructions that the patient is willing to accept.
9. Document the specifics of the encounter with the patient in their medical record. Include information on the patient's decision-making capacity, the specific advantages of your recommended treatment versus the risks of leaving the hospital, your efforts to persuade the patient to stay, and your compassionate commitment to their potential return for any reason. Ensure the patient signs an AMA form covering these details, witnessed by a family member or staff member.
10. Do not concern yourself, in private hospitals, with whether the patient's insurance will deny payment if they choose to leave. Their insurance coverage is not your responsibility, but a malpractice lawsuit would certainly become your concern.

It is crucial for the inter-professional healthcare team to be well versed in patient rights and ethical considerations. Every physician, nurse, and allied health provider should strive to deliver care in accordance with these principles. This approach enhances the likelihood of achieving optimal medical outcomes while minimising the potential for legal or ethical repercussions.

As previously mentioned, the practice of shared decision-making is a valuable tool for both patients and healthcare team members to incorporate various elements of patient rights. Collaborative decision-making helps strike a balance between two extremes: paternalism, where the patient has no input, and overwhelming the patient with information and choices, leaving them to decide without proper clinical guidance. When employed appropriately, shared decision-making can promote patient rights such as beneficence, non-maleficence, patient autonomy, patient-provider trust, and more. It serves to clarify patient goals for both the patient and the healthcare team, a trend that continues to gain support through ongoing research.

Shared decision-making, coupled with decision aids, led to patients feeling more informed, knowledgeable, and better aligned with their values. Patients also developed a more accurate understanding of risks and actively participated in decision-making. Moreover, other studies have demonstrated the effectiveness of shared decision-making across various medical specialties. For instance, in the treatment of depression in primary care, this approach resulted in improved treatment outcomes and higher patient satisfaction without prolonging consultation times. Numerous studies across different specialties and healthcare settings have consistently shown positive results regarding the efficacy of shared decision-making. By implementing this approach and other ethical best practices while fostering ongoing education, healthcare providers and team members can actively promote patient rights and improve overall outcomes [6–8].

Guidance by ethical principles and respect for patient rights should serve as the foundation for all patient interactions. While there is no formal legal framework at the national level in North America, many individual states and provinces have developed their own specific policies regarding patient rights. In regions where such policies are lacking, it becomes the responsibility of individual healthcare institutions to decide whether to implement their own systems. Failure to adhere to ethical and legal standards can result in patient dissatisfaction, potential medical malpractice claims, and the risk of losing clinical privileges or a medical license. Key areas that demand attention include patient competence, consent, the right to refuse treatment, emergency care, confidentiality, and the continuity of care.

A proper understanding of ethical principles and their application to specific situations is essential across all clinical specialties and healthcare settings. Without a comprehensive grasp of patient rights, healthcare teams may inadvertently exhibit behaviours that undermine patient autonomy. This can manifest in various ways, such as excessively paternalistic actions or making decisions on behalf of the patient or their family. Additionally, there may be instances where not all treatment options, risks, or side effects are adequately disclosed. Ethical questions arise when providers choose to omit certain details based on their perception of low likelihood or clinical judgment. While this approach may be perceived as time-saving or in the patient's best interest, it raises concerns about whether patients are genuinely fully informed or merely sufficiently informed. This challenge can occur in urgent situations with limited time, as well as in end-of-life decisions where families may not fully comprehend the extent of certain treatment options. Although failure to respect patient autonomy is just one example, it underscores the importance of upholding all patient rights. By fostering open communication with patients regarding their care goals, engaging in shared decision-making, and possessing a comprehensive understanding of patient rights, healthcare teams can minimise the risk of infringing upon these rights in various healthcare settings [7, 8].

References

1. Chapman CB, Stratton VS. Swanlond: the fourteenth-century ancestor of the law of malpractice. Pharos Alpha Omega Alpha Honor Med Soc. 1982;45(4):20–4.
2. Olejarczyk JP, Young M. Patient rights and ethics. [Updated 2022 Nov 28]. In: StatPearls [Internet]. Treasure Island: StatPearls Publishing.
3. Emanuel EJ, Emanuel LL. Four models of the physician-patient relationship. JAMA. 1992;267(16):2221–6.
4. Physician and patient; or a practical view of the mutual duties, relations, and interests of the medical profession and the community. Br Foreign Med Chir Rev. 1850;5(12):503–10.
5. International code of medical ethics (World Medical Associaion, London, October 1949). Madjalah Kedokt Indones. 1959;9:462.
6. Stacey D, Légaré F, Lewis K, Barry MJ, Bennett CL, Eden KB, Holmes-Rovner M, Llewellyn-Thomas H, Lyddiatt A, Thomson R, Trevena L. Decision aids for people facing health treatment or screening decisions. Cochrane Database Syst Rev. 2017;4(4):CD001431.
7. Loh A, Simon D, Wills CE, Kriston L, Niebling W, Härter M. The effects of a shared decision-making intervention in primary care of depression: a cluster-randomized controlled trial. Patient Educ Couns. 2007;67(3):324–32.
8. Wilson CD, Probe RA. Shared decision-making in Orthopaedic surgery. J Am Acad Orthop Surg. 2020;28(23):e1032–41.

Chapter 15
The Conflict Between Autonomy and Beneficence

The autonomy model of clinical decision-making, rooted in the principles of individual dignity and human rights, emphasises privacy, self-determination, and informed decision-making. This model, which has gained prominence in recent decades, challenges the traditional paternalistic approach where physicians make decisions on behalf of patients without their active involvement.

Voltaire once stated that "the art of medicine consists in amusing the patient while nature cures the disease." However, he also recognised that those who work together with skill and compassion to restore health to others hold a special place in society. This group includes not only healthcare professionals but also philosophers, historians, writers, artists, performers, and social scientists, all of whom contribute their expertise and humanity to promote healing in others.

The origins of the autonomy model can be traced back to the Enlightenment era, with its focus on individual rights and freedoms. However, it took time for these principles to influence the medical field, where paternalism had long been the norm. The shift towards patient autonomy gained momentum due to several factors, including the expansion of democracy, improved public education, and greater awareness of medical advances and ethical issues. These changes led to a growing desire among the public to participate in decisions about their healthcare. People began to understand that medical choices often involved not only scientific expertise but also personal values and ethical considerations. While there were sporadic historical instances of patient involvement in medical decisions, paternalism remained dominant for most of medical history. In the past, factors such as a wide knowledge gap between physicians and patients, lack of medical alternatives, and the quasi-hieratic power attributed to physicians contributed to the acceptance of paternalism [1].

However, in modern times, medical advancements have given healthcare professionals unprecedented power to influence individual lives. Patients, now better educated and more informed, realise the significance of the decisions made by doctors and their moral and ethical implications. While the professionalisation of medicine has brought many benefits, it has also led to certain issues, such as the perception of

S. Abbas, *Medical Ethics*, https://doi.org/10.1007/978-981-96-9199-9_15

physicians as a superior class and a sense of condescension in doctor-patient relationships. These factors have fuelled the patient autonomy movement, as people seek to protect their values and rights in the face of medical decisions that touch on deeply held beliefs. It is important to note that while the autonomy model challenges paternalism, it does not dismiss it entirely. There are situations where physicians must make decisions based on their expertise and intuition, especially when dealing with uncertain diagnoses or treatments. However, in such cases, clear communication of uncertainties and shared decision-making can help balance autonomy and beneficence. Ultimately, the autonomy model represents a significant shift in medical ethics, emphasising the importance of respecting patients' rights, values, and decisions while recognising the complexities of healthcare decision-making in the real world [2].

Patient autonomy in medical decision-making is a fundamental principle, but it has certain limitations that must be considered:

1. Context Limitations: The application of the autonomy model may not be suitable in all medical contexts. In some situations, such as when dealing with senile or incapacitated patients or in emergencies, paternalism may be more appropriate to ensure the patient's best interests. The clinical context can change rapidly, affecting the moral defensibility of paternalism or autonomy. It is essential to assess each case individually while respecting patient autonomy when possible [2].
2. Existential Limitations: The impact of illness: Illness and disease can significantly impact a patient's autonomy. The effects of illness, pain, fear, and the clinical environment can disrupt self-direction, life plans, deliberation, and decision-making. While most patients retain their autonomy to some extent, it is crucial to acknowledge that becoming a patient can modify the autonomy model significantly.
3. Conceptual Limitations as a Model: The autonomy model is just one of several ethical norms governing the doctor–patient relationship. Other formulations, such as restoring autonomy, safeguarding the person, respecting persons, healing, prioritising patient needs, making good medical decisions, or acting in the patient's best interests, can offer different perspectives on the physician's obligations. These various formulations recognise that medical ethics encompasses a range of principles and cannot be reduced to a strict dichotomy between autonomy and paternalism.

While patient autonomy is a vital ethical principle in medicine, it must be considered within the context of the patient's condition, the impact of illness, and the complexity of the doctor–patient relationship. Medical ethics should account for the variability of clinical situations and recognise that different formulations of ethical norms may apply depending on the circumstances [3].

Main Dimensions

(a) Non-Maleficence: Physicians must avoid causing harm to patients. The famous Hippocratic principle "First, do no harm" encapsulates this aspect of beneficence. It emphasises the importance of not causing additional suffering or damage to the patient.
(b) Beneficence as Positively Promoting Good: Beyond merely avoiding harm, beneficence also entails actively promoting the well-being and good health of patients. This involves diagnosing and treating illnesses, alleviating suffering, and improving the overall quality of life for patients.

Patient-Centredness: Beneficence in medicine is fundamentally patient-centred. It requires that physicians act in the best interests of their patients, considering their individual values, preferences, and goals. This patient-centred approach acknowledges the uniqueness of each patient's situation.

1. Trust and Reciprocity: The beneficence model emphasises trust and reciprocity between the physician and the patient. Patients trust physicians to act in their best interests, and in return, they provide information, consent, and cooperation necessary for effective diagnosis and treatment. This trust is essential for the therapeutic relationship to function optimally.
2. Shared Decision-Making: While beneficence recognises the physician's expertise, it also values the patient's autonomy and participation in medical decisions. Physicians and patients should engage in shared decision-making, where the physician provides information, recommendations, and options, and the patient makes informed choices based on their values and preferences.
3. Respect for Autonomy: The beneficence model respects and upholds the autonomy of patients. It recognises that patients have the right to make decisions about their own bodies and health, even if those decisions may not align with the physician's recommendations. Physicians should support patients in making autonomous choices, as long as those choices do not lead to harm to themselves or others.
4. Ethical Considerations: In the beneficence model, ethical considerations are crucial. Physicians must navigate complex ethical issues, balancing the principles of beneficence, non-maleficence, autonomy, and justice. Ethical dilemmas may arise when patient values and medical recommendations conflict, and careful ethical reasoning is required to resolve such dilemmas.
5. Continual Assessment and Improvement: Beneficence also encourages a commitment to continual assessment and improvement in medical practice. Physicians should strive to enhance their knowledge and skills to better serve the interests of their patients. This includes staying up-to-date with medical advancements and ethical standards [4, 5].

The beneficence model in medicine emphasises the physician's duty to promote the well-being of patients while respecting their autonomy and fostering trust and collaboration. It recognises the multifaceted nature of beneficence, encompassing both the avoidance of harm and the active pursuit of good, all within the context of a patient-centred and ethical approach to healthcare.

Beneficence is a central requirement in the field of medicine, encompassing three distinct obligations. First, the paramount concern of a physician should be the patient's problems and needs, typically taking precedence over all other considerations, except in the rarest of circumstances. Second, the avoidance of harm is imperative, as a physician cannot fulfil their promise to help if they intentionally harm the patient for any reason. Third, the principles of autonomy and paternalism should yield to the obligation to act beneficently. In other words, the choice between promoting autonomy or acting paternalistically should be based on what best serves the patient's interests, rather than the physician's personal beliefs or emotional impulses.

Another hallmark of the beneficence model is the prioritisation of the patient's existential condition over traditional professional codes. For instance, when determining the limits of autonomy for a seriously ill patient, factors such as the patient's ability to make rational decisions, their values, age, the nature of the illness, the physician's values, and the clinical setting should be considered. These factors reflect the patient's personal condition, while others pertain to the healthcare professional and the environment.

Unlike models that emphasise the automatic supremacy of a single value, such as patient autonomy or medical paternalism, the beneficence model does not impose a predefined hierarchy of values. Each patient must be approached individually, with decisions made based on what serves their best interests. This approach necessitates the identification, ranking, discussion, and negotiation of values by both patients and physicians, focusing on the unique good of each patient while recognising that general ethical principles applicable to multiple patients remain valid [6, 7].

Consensus-building is another integral aspect of the beneficence model. Since values should not be imposed, and decisions should involve the active participation of patients and healthcare team members, consensus is crucial. Although reaching a consensus may require time and effort, it helps prevent later conflicts during the course of a serious illness. Unlike models that offer simplified decision-making mechanisms, the beneficence model encourages ongoing dialogue and mutual exchange between doctors and patients while respecting their moral agency.

The beneficence model incorporates a prudential moral objective, aiming to resolve complex ethical dilemmas while preserving as many values as possible for both patients and physicians. While this may not be the sole goal of bioethics, it aligns with a patient-oriented, consensus-driven approach in which prudential judgments are made on a case-by-case basis.

Lastly, the beneficence model relies on explicit axioms to guide ethical decision-making. These axioms, necessary to avoid moral pitfalls present in other models, include principles such as the freedom of both doctor and patient to make informed decisions and act as moral agents, the physician's responsibility to provide information and protect the vulnerable, the importance of the physician's personal moral integrity, and the need to address moral ambiguity without abandoning the search for what is right and good in each decision.

The beneficence model reconciles the values of patient welfare and patient autonomy, recognising that they need not be in perpetual conflict for medicine to fulfil its healing mission. It emphasises the importance of beneficence as a guiding principle in medicine, taking into account the ethical tradition of individuals united in community rather than emphasising autonomous individualism [9, 10].

Families often get involved in the decision making which could impinge on patient's own autonomy and agency, some times if the condition is complex and the decision is difficult the following strategy is advised:

Strategies and Examples.
Avoid Overreacting.
Listen Actively.
Try to understand if the patient's concern is driven by their own fears or distress.
Determine if their request arises from a sense of responsibility and manage their concerns.
Show Understanding.
Express empathy by acknowledging their love and concern for the patient.
Recognise their desire to protect the patient from harm.
Share Empathy.
Align with the family's goal of safeguarding the patient's well-being.
Express your commitment to doing everything possible for the patient's welfare.
Emphasise the importance of truthfulness, not only as a physician but as a fellow human being.
Offer Constructive Suggestions.
Foster Open Communication.

When discussing the patient's preferences, remember that revealing the diagnosis is not always necessary.

Consider utilising professional medical interpreters for improved communication for patients who speak different languages.

Provide access to support services like chaplaincy, social work, and patient representatives to assist both the patient and the family during this challenging period.

Understand the patient's desired level of involvement in decision-making or if they prefer to defer to the family [8, 9, 11].

References

1. Newton S. The patient as responsible adult: consequences of the revised perspective. In: Proceedings of the Fifty-Fifth Annual Business Meeting of the American Psychological Association; 1982. p. 240–49.
2. Pellegrino ED. Foreword to T. Percival, The ethics beneath the etiquette. In: Medical ethics, or, a code of institutes and precepts, adapted to the professional conduct of physicians and surgeons. 1985.
3. Thomasma DC. Professional and ethical obligations toward the aged. Linacre Q. 1981;48:12.
4. Soffer A. Searching questions and inappropriate answers. Chest. 1982;81:533.

5. Beauchamp T, Childress J. Principles of biomedical ethics. Edicoes Loyola; 1979. p. 56–7.
6. McGovern. The patient comes first. F Med. 1980;3:596–98.
7. Pellegrino ED. The healing relationship: architectonics of clinical medicine. In: IV The clinical encounter: the moral fabric of the patient-physician relationship, The Phil. & Med. Book Series E. Shelp ed. 1983.
8. Thomasma CD, Pellegrino ED. Philosophy of medicine as the source for medical ethics. Metamed. 1981;2:5–11.
9. Siegler M. Critical illness: The limits of autonomy, 7 Hastings Center Report. 12 Oct. 1977.
10. Ackerman TF. What bioethics should be. J Med Philos. 1980;5:260.
11. Scharf A, Voigt L, Vardhana S, Matsoukas K, Wall LM, Arevalo M, Diamond LC. What should clinicians do when a patient's autonomy undermines her being treated equitably? AMA J Ethics. 2021;23(2):E97–108. https://doi.org/10.1001/amajethics.2021.97. PMID: 33635189; PMCID: PMC8366686.

Chapter 16
Moral and Ethical Guidance for Medical Students

Modern medical practice is a complex and dynamic field that demands healthcare professionals to integrate various elements effectively. This integration involves the harmonious blending of knowledge, skills, and wisdom to deliver the best possible care that aligns with the unique requirements of each patient, their specific context, and the available resources at hand.

First, knowledge forms the foundation of medical practice. It encompasses the vast and ever-expanding body of information, research findings, and clinical data that underpin the practice of medicine. This knowledge base informs the diagnostic and treatment decisions made by healthcare providers, ensuring that they are evidence-based and aligned with the best practices established by the medical community.

Second, skills are essential in translating knowledge into action. Medical professionals must possess a diverse set of clinical and technical skills to effectively diagnose, treat, and manage a wide range of medical conditions. These skills include everything from conducting physical examinations and performing surgical procedures to interpreting diagnostic tests and prescribing appropriate medications. Proficiency in these skills allows healthcare providers to deliver precise and effective care, contributing to better patient outcomes.

However, beyond knowledge and skills, wisdom plays a crucial role in modern medical practice. Wisdom in medicine extends beyond textbook learning and clinical techniques. It encompasses the ability to make sound moral judgments in the face of complex ethical dilemmas. Healthcare professionals often encounter situations where they must balance competing interests, such as patient autonomy, beneficence, and resource allocation. In such instances, wisdom guides them to make ethically sound decisions that prioritise the well-being of the patient while respecting the broader constraints of the healthcare system.

In essence, the synthesis of knowledge, skills, and wisdom is the hallmark of a competent and compassionate healthcare provider. It ensures that patients receive care that is not only medically accurate but also ethically grounded. By harmonising these elements, healthcare professionals can navigate the intricacies of modern

S. Abbas, *Medical Ethics*, https://doi.org/10.1007/978-981-96-9199-9_16

medicine, making choices that promote the best possible outcomes for their patients while upholding the highest moral standards of their profession.

The increasing focus on knowledge, techniques, and evidence-based medicine in medical education has raised concerns about its potential impact on the doctor-patient relationship. Medical education is becoming more aware of this issue and is emphasising the development of interpersonal skills, professional behaviours, and attitudes, as well as the personal growth and well-being of medical students.

Approximately 15% of physicians may experience impairment during their careers. Impairment goes beyond diagnostic errors and inappropriate treatment and can include avoidance of patients' psychological needs, dehumanised care, and boundary violations. Substance abuse is also a concern, with around 1% of doctors abusing opiates and up to 7–8% having significant alcohol problems. These issues can have serious implications for patient care.

Depression is prevalent among medical professionals, with about 23% of interns, residents, and fellows experiencing some degree of depression. Doctors often have negative attitudes about mental disorders, attempt to self-treat, and are reluctant to seek help. Depression is a leading cause of suicide among doctors, particularly among younger female physicians.

Some personality characteristics, such as competitiveness, high self-expectations, rigidity, and an excessive concern for detail, may contribute to doctors' vulnerability to personal strain and professional impairment. Medical training, which emphasises excessive devotion to work and often lacks positive reinforcement, can compound these problems.

Medical students frequently witness unethical practices and may be subjected to mistreatment, including verbal abuse, intimidation, and harassment. This raises questions about the fairness of holding students to high professional standards when faculty behaviour sometimes falls short.

Medical education is addressing the challenges posed by the increasing emphasis on knowledge and evidence-based medicine, with a focus on developing students' interpersonal skills and well-being. However, issues such as impairment, substance abuse, depression, and mistreatment in medical training continue to be significant concerns for the profession [1, 2].

Main Considerations

In the realm of medical practice, there exists a moral responsibility for medical education to prioritise the awareness, prevention, and mitigation of critical issues. Such an emphasis not only benefits doctors but also the patients under their care and the broader community. Surprisingly, the assessment of non-cognitive attributes and professionalism in medical students has not garnered the same level of attention as the evaluation of clinical competence, knowledge, and technical skills. Moreover, the development, publication, and evaluation of strategies for assessing professional and unprofessional behaviours in medical schools remain limited.

Assessment serves as a vital means through which medical institutions communicate the importance of specific domains of study, and the absence of formal assessment can diminish the impact of teaching efforts. Objectives that lack rigorous testing tend to be perceived as less significant, regardless of their actual importance, as indicated by educators and reports. A medical school that neglects such assessment covertly undermines the cultivation of attitudes related to personal and professional development across its curriculum.

Nonetheless, a significant challenge in the assessment process lies in the hesitation of physicians to directly address problem behaviours, often opting for indirect responses that avoid moral language. This reluctance to confront underlying attitudes leaves students or junior doctors susceptible to misinterpreting, undervaluing, or altogether missing subtle feedback. Additionally, students in clinical years may face the challenge of undergoing multiple short rotations, with each clinical rotation potentially neglecting ownership of the realm of professional competency.

In conjunction with assessment, it is imperative to establish well-defined processes for addressing unsatisfactory performance, offering opportunities for active remediation and, when necessary, considering professional disqualification before graduation. This is underscored in Ratzan's review of "Blind Eye: How the Medical Establishment Let a Doctor Get Away with Murder, which recounts the chilling story of a suspected medical serial killer in Southern Illinois." [3–5]

When clinicians are compelled to evaluate the behaviour of their peers, they are naturally prompted to reflect on their own performance. This influence on education can be even more profound than the impact of specific courses.

Aspects of Professional Behaviour

Assessment

For professional behaviours and attitudes with significant consequences, such as the potential to withhold education, valid, reliable, and acceptable assessment tools, and procedures are imperative.

Timing of Assessment

Many experts advocate initiating assessments early in the curriculum for several reasons.

Expelling students from advanced clerkships due to inadequate behaviour is challenging when introduced late in the curriculum.

Inadequate professional behaviour often surfaces during the early stages of medical training.

Time is needed for remediation and review if inadequate behaviour is to be addressed.

Reliable assessment necessitates repeated observations.

Serial observations over an extended period help counter faculty's reluctance to provide negative evaluations.

Identified students can potentially benefit from monitoring and placement in structured clerkship sites with selected faculty who can assist them with specific professionalism issues [6].

Assessment Strategies in Use

Various medical schools have embraced the active promotion of professionalism, employing diverse evaluation methods and consequences. Some have developed specific evaluation tools and procedures akin to assessing academic skills.

Attendance Records: Some institutions resort to superficial evaluations such as tracking attendance or participation. However, this approach fails to adequately focus on curricular content and may exacerbate the perceived disparities in importance between professionalism and basic sciences or clinical skills, which receive more rigorous evaluation [7, 8].

Self and Peer Assessment: At certain schools, students evaluate both themselves and their peers concerning professional attitudes and behaviour. While some students may find this process uncomfortable, it helps foster honest self-assessment. However, accurate self-assessment can be challenging to achieve, prompting some to argue that for summative assessment, the focus should remain on actual clinical behaviour.

Patient Evaluations: Patient opinions are considered by some as the "gold standard" for assessing the humanistic attributes of physicians. Recent research suggests that, within a controlled context and through aggregated opinions, patients can provide reliable and valid global assessments that contribute to the evaluation of a student's clinical skills [8].

Observation of Behaviours: Behavioural observations may involve various observers, including teachers, psychologists, peers, nursing staff, and simulated patients. Repeated observations by different assessors are necessary to reliably evaluate actual behaviour. Nurses' assessments appear to closely align with those of patients, indicating that nurses' evaluations could enhance reliability.

Student Journals: Some institutions base assessment on student journal entries, which include reactions to set topics, the quality of class discussions, and essay examinations.

Psychological Tests: Psychological tests measuring maturity, responsibility, self-control, tolerance, self-acceptance, and flexibility have been proposed as evaluation tools. Questionnaires assessing changes in attitudes toward psychosocial aspects of medicine, tolerance of ambiguity, empathy, well-being, stress, burnout, and self-esteem have also been suggested.

Structured Examinations: In some institutions, themes like health law and ethics are assessed using methods such as the modified essay question (MEQ) and the Objective Structured Clinical Examination (OSCE) to directly evaluate professional values, attitudes, and interaction skills. These methods aim to assess not only what students know but also what they can do in an unobserved work context [8–11].

Various international medical schools have documented the processes and instruments they employ for non-cognitive evaluation, although the level of detail varies.

Medical Education Assesses

Interpersonal Skills: How students interact with peers, staff, and patients.

Self-Reflection: Students' ability to reflect on actions and behaviours.

Evaluating students' communication skills.

Assessing empathy, respect, responsibility, and task efficiency.

Self-care promotion is not a focus of these assessments.

University of California, San Francisco School of Medicine.

This school has a comprehensive evaluation system where students are assessed in clinical rotations. Ratings range from 1 (excellent) to 4 (problem) for knowledge, clinical skills, and interpersonal skills. A "concern" or "problem" rating in interpersonal skills triggers a Psychiatric Evaluation Form, leading to a school review.

Unprofessional Behavior:

Between 1995 and 1998, 29 unprofessional behaviour reports on 24 students were submitted. Issues included unmet professional responsibility, poor relationships with the health team, resistance to feedback, arrogance, and inadequate patient rapport. Some students were referred for counselling, but most graduated with professionalism concerns in residency recommendations.

1. Disparity in Reporting

   Team dynamics and professionalism may influence reporting patterns.
2. Student Support and Feedback

   Student support is crucial for the evaluation system's success. The liaison committee recommended recording student agreement or disagreement with evaluations, obtaining student signatures, and recording counselling sessions.
3. Faculty Concerns

   Some preclinical faculty feel they lack sufficient contact with students to evaluate professionalism effectively.

Graduates were affected by the strike. University of California graduates are assessed after their postgraduate years for academic skills, attitudes, and behaviours. "Attitudes" are a common reason for residency failures.

Piaget and Kohlberg are notable figures in the study of moral judgment development, and their work forms the foundation of our current understanding in this field. Researchers have conducted quantitative longitudinal studies that utilise standardised tests based on Kohlberg's theory to investigate how moral development unfolds during medical education.

One such study conducted by Lind's group compared medical students with students in other tertiary educational programs. Surprisingly, the findings revealed a decline in moral judgment competence among medical students, whereas their peers in other programs exhibited the expected growth in moral judgment typical of early adulthood. Additional research studies have corroborated these findings, highlighting a regression in moral judgment among medical students, particularly coinciding with their exposure to clinical settings.

As medical students progress through their training, a noticeable shift occurs in their approach to moral judgment. They tend to prioritise pleasing others over adhering to social justice imperatives, representing a retrograde movement towards what Kohlberg referred to as a conventional rather than a post-conventional level of moral reasoning.

Furthermore, some studies have uncovered the phenomenon of moral segmentation among medical students. This means that as their training advances, medical students tend to apply a lower level of moral reasoning when faced with moral dilemmas in clinical settings compared to non-clinical contexts. These findings shed light on the complex interplay between medical education and moral development, revealing intriguing shifts and nuances in the moral judgment of future healthcare professionals [12–14].

The modern clinical setting is complex and dynamic, with relationships and system processes that are interspersed by critical events. The students' experiences showed a sharp contrast between the reality of clinical practice and the explicitly taught professionalism ideals. The incongruence between what the students experience and their ideals led to distress-provoked early confusion followed by defensiveness. Students become caught in what Baxter Magolda refers to as the "crossroads space," with tension and uncertainty as they attempt to reconcile new experiences with an emerging identity and belief system. This disequilibrium is described as a necessary stage and driver towards self-authorship. Identity development according to DST is characterised by cycles of commitment (identity) and exploration for solutions.

During this uncertain period, students faced a dilemma and adopted two primary coping mechanisms: desensitisation and justification. Some became emotionally insensitive as a means of self-protection, while others justified the behaviours of their superiors. This justification indicated a growing identification with their senior colleagues and an acknowledgment of the complexities and competing priorities in healthcare.

Additionally, some students tried to rationalise their own actions, deviating from their ideals. Their main goal was simply to navigate through their training, complete their requirements, and persevere. Many students harboured feelings of disappointment in their training, particularly regarding the perceived lack of support they had received. These students strongly advocated for more opportunities to discuss their experiences in clinical settings and for education in assertiveness and ethical reasoning [14–16].

Medical educators must ensure safe and stimulating learning environments for students. Role models, whether positive or negative, significantly shape student values, motivations, and behaviours. Toxic healthcare settings are detrimental to both patient care and the well-being of medical students. Students and junior medical officers must be empowered to speak out against unprofessional behaviours, requiring the confidence and means to act on their moral judgments. This cross-sectional study included three years of a medical cohort, enabling a comparison of perspectives across different stages of training. Future research should investigate the moral development of young graduates as they progress in their careers and explore intervention effectiveness on medical student experiences and moral growth [17].

Examples of poor moral behaviour:

1. Cheating and Plagiarism

   Cheating in exams
   Signing absent peers into classes
   Claiming others' work as your own
   Sharing exam questions with fellow students
   Forging supervisor signatures or feedback

2. Dishonesty and Fraud

   Falsifying research
   Committing financial fraud
   Creating fraudulent documents like CVs
   Misrepresenting qualifications
   Not disclosing misconduct issues to the school
   Withholding or misrepresenting health conditions

3. Misconduct and Substance Use

   Driving under the influence
   Misusing prescription medication
   Alcohol or drug use affecting work or education
   Dealing, possessing, or supplying drugs
   Excessive alcohol consumption
   Aggressive, violent, or threatening behaviour

4. Failure to Demonstrate Good Medical Practice

   Misusing social media
   Breaching patient confidentiality
   Misleading patients about care
   Inadequate consent procedures
   Harassment
   Inappropriate examinations or boundary violations
   Unlawful discrimination

5. Persistent Inappropriate Behaviour

Lack of commitment or engagement
Poor time management
Weak communication skills
Ignoring educational advice and feedback
Rudeness to patients, colleagues, or others
Disruptive behaviour in teaching or training
Challenging clinical teachers or refusing criticism
Failing to respond to communications
Non-attendance
Neglecting administrative tasks [18].

References

1. Novack DH, Epstein RM, Paulsen RH. Toward creating physician healers: fostering medical students' self awareness, personal growth and well-being. Acad Med. 1999;74:516–20.
2. Lawrence JM. The impaired doctor. Med J Aust. 1992;157:4–6.
3. Papadakis MA, Osborn EHS, Cooke M, et al. A strategy for the detection and evaluation of unprofessional behaviour in medical students. Acad Med. 1999;74:980–90.
4. Goldie J, Schwartz L, McConnachie A, et al. The impact of three years' ethics teaching, in an integrated medical curriculum, on students' proposed behaviour on meeting ethical dilemmas. Med Educ. 2002;36:489–97.
5. Burack JH, Irby DM, Carline JD, et al. Teaching compassion and respect. Attending physicians' responses to problematic behaviours. J Gen Intern Med. 1999;14:49–55.
6. Van Luijk SJ, Smeets JGE, Wolfhagen I, et al. Assessing professional behaviour and the role of academic advice at the Maastricht Medical School. Med Teacher. 2000;22:68–172.
7. Miller GD, Frank D, Franks RD, et al. Noncognitive criteria for assessing students in North American medical schools. Acad Med. 1989;42:42–5.
8. Makoul G, Curry RH, Novack DH. The future of medical school courses in professional skills and perspectives. Acad Med. 1998;73:48–51.
9. Woollicroft JO, Howell JD, Patel BP, et al. Resident-patient interactions: the humanistic qualities of internal medicine residents assessed by patients, attending physicians, program supervisors and nurses. Acad Med. 1994;69:216–24.
10. Mitchell KR, Myser C, Kerridge IH. Assessing the clinical ethical competence of undergraduate medical students. J Med Ethics. 1993;19:230–6.
11. Blake JM, Norman GR, Smith EKM. Report card from McMaster: student evaluation at a problem-based medical school. Lancet. 1995;345:899–901.
12. Whetnall EM. The moral judgment of the child. By Jean Piaget. (International library of psychology and philosophy. London: Kegan Paul, Trench, Trübner & Co. 1932. ix + 417. Price 12s. 6d). Philosophy. 1933;8(31):373–4.
13. Kohlberg L, Hersh RH. Moral development: a review of the theory. Theory Pract. 1977;16(2):53–9.
14. Lind G. Moral regression in medical students and their learning environment. Revista Brasileira de Educacao Médica. 2000;24(3):24–33.
15. Magolda M. The evolution of self-authorship. In: Khine MS, editor. Knowing, knowledge and beliefs. Chicago: Springer; 2010.
16. Pizzolato JE. Creating crossroads for self-authorship: investigating the provocative moment. J Coll Stud Dev. 2005;46(6):624–41.

17. Rotenstein LS, Ramos MA, Torre M, Segal JB, Peluso MJ, Guille C, et al. Prevalence of depression, depressive symptoms, and suicidal ideation among medical students: a systematic review and meta-analysis. JAMA. 2016;316(21):2214–36.
18. https://www.gmc-uk.org/education/standards-guidance-and-curricula/guidance/student-professionalism-and-ftp/professional-behaviour-and-fitness-to-practise/table-1-reasons-for-impaired-fitness-to-practise-in-medical-students

Chapter 17
Decision-Making

"Knowledge is power", Francis Bacon, the philosopher of the industrial revolution.

Patient-centred care involves acknowledging diverse perspectives and building strong therapeutic relationships to improve patient outcomes. Knowledge can be sourced from various avenues, including:

1. Facts and Figures: This involves utilising measurements, numerical data, and statistics, often found in evidence-based research.
2. Observation and Empirical Thought: Knowledge can be gained by recognising patterns and making direct measurements using one's own senses. The scientific method heavily relies on this approach.
3. Experience: Past personal experiences, even if anecdotal, shape what we consider to be true. While not always valued in evidence-based medicine, anecdotal evidence can be influential.
4. Hands-On Learning (Heuristics): Knowledge can be acquired through practical, hands-on experience. For example, knowing how to perform a medical procedure based on previous learning.
5. Learning from Others: Gathering information from various sources, including experts, books, education, media, and advertising. Social connections and affiliations also contribute to our understanding of truth, as does cultural and traditional knowledge.
6. Narratives and Art: Stories and artistic expressions are powerful tools for conveying knowledge and have been used throughout history to inform future generations.
7. Instinct and Personality: Sometimes, individuals simply know something based on their instincts or personal characteristics.
8. Intuition and Inspiration: In the realm of conventional medicine, intuition and inspiration can play a role in diagnosis and treatment decisions.
9. Serendipity, Chance, Luck: Occasionally, important discoveries or knowledge emerge from unexpected or chance occurrences.

S. Abbas, *Medical Ethics*, https://doi.org/10.1007/978-981-96-9199-9_17

10. Collective Consciousness: Some believe that knowledge can spread across a group when one member develops it, contributing to collective understanding.
11. Contemplation and Reflection: Mindful awareness and intentional reflection, using various methods or traditions, can enhance one's understanding of different subjects.
12. Spiritual and Personal Means: Personal beliefs and spirituality can also be a significant source of knowledge, often on deeply personal matters.

These diverse sources of knowledge highlight the complexity of how individuals come to understand and perceive truth in various aspects of life, including healthcare.

Knowledge comes from observation, reason, and trust in information from others (trust is pivotal to human society), all these are fallible. In the field of medicine decision-making is pivoted on knowledge, understanding the concepts of "knowing that," "knowing how," and "tacit knowledge" which build the launching pad for a scientific argument that is essential for healthcare professionals to make a decision where any conclusion should have a link to a "factual premise."

Knowing that (Declarative Knowledge)

What It Is: "Knowing that" refers to explicit or declarative knowledge, which involves understanding and being able to express facts, information, concepts, and principles. This knowledge can typically be articulated and transferred through language, textbooks, lectures, or written documentation.

Application in Medicine: In medicine, "knowing that" includes knowledge of anatomical structures, physiological processes, medical terminology, diagnostic criteria, medical guidelines, and factual information. It involves having a grasp of the theoretical and academic aspects of healthcare.

Knowing How (Procedural Knowledge)

What It Is: "Knowing how" relates to practical or procedural knowledge. It involves the ability to apply theoretical knowledge to perform specific tasks, procedures, or skills. This knowledge often requires hands-on experience and the development of clinical expertise.

Application in Medicine: In healthcare, "knowing how" encompasses clinical skills, diagnostic abilities, surgical techniques, and medical procedures. Healthcare professionals, such as surgeons, nurses, and therapists, must have the practical skills and proficiency to perform their roles effectively.

Tacit Knowledge

What It Is: Tacit knowledge is a form of knowledge that is challenging to express explicitly through language or formalised documentation. It's deeply rooted in personal experience, intuition, and the practical aspects of a profession. Tacit knowledge is often developed through observation, experience, and a deep understanding of complex, real-world situations.

Application in Medicine: In medicine, tacit knowledge is crucial for clinical decision-making, patient care, and developing the "art of medicine." It includes skills like clinical judgment, patient interaction, adaptability in complex and uncertain situations, and the ability to integrate various sources of information. Tacit knowledge allows healthcare professionals to navigate the intricate and unpredictable aspects of patient care effectively.

Healthcare professionals require a combination of "knowing that," "knowing how," and tacit knowledge to provide comprehensive and effective patient care. While "knowing that" is the foundation of theoretical knowledge, "knowing how" represents practical and procedural skills, and tacit knowledge enables professionals to apply their expertise to real-world clinical scenarios. These different forms of knowledge complement each other and contribute to the development of competent and compassionate healthcare practitioners [1].

Any conclusion made is vulnerable to "fallibilism" as no argument is stronger than its weakest link.

Decisions Are Made by Following Concepts

A. Inductive Inference: In medicine refers to a process of drawing general conclusions or making predictions based on specific observations, data, or evidence gathered from clinical or research experiences. In this context, it involves reasoning from individual cases or specific pieces of information to create broader generalisations, theories, or diagnostic conclusions.

   Here are some key points about inductive inference in medicine:

   1. Observation and Data Collection: Inductive reasoning begins with the collection of specific data or observations in a clinical or research setting. These observations may include patient symptoms, laboratory results, medical histories, and other relevant information.
   2. Pattern Recognition: Medical professionals and researchers look for patterns, trends, or recurring characteristics within the collected data. They aim to identify commonalities or correlations among different cases or pieces of information.
   3. Generalisation: Based on the identified patterns or commonalities, inductive inference involves making general statements or hypotheses about a broader population or a class of medical conditions. It moves from specific instances to more general conclusions.

4. Diagnostic Reasoning: In clinical medicine, inductive inference plays a significant role in diagnostic reasoning. Physicians often encounter patients with symptoms that may not fit a textbook description of a known condition. They use inductive reasoning to diagnose patients by recognising patterns of symptoms and signs.
5. Research and Evidence-Based Medicine: In research, inductive inference is essential for generating hypotheses and theories based on empirical data. It contributes to the development of new medical knowledge, treatment approaches, and guidelines.
6. Uncertainty: It is important to note that inductive inference comes with a degree of uncertainty. Generalisations and hypotheses drawn through this process are based on probability and may not always hold true for every case.
7. Confirmation and Testing: Once generalisations are made through inductive inference, they often need to be confirmed and tested through further research, experimentation, or clinical trials to establish their validity.

Inductive inference complements deductive reasoning in medicine, where deductive reasoning involves starting with general principles or theories and applying them to specific cases. Inductive inference is a valuable tool for physicians, researchers, and healthcare professionals as they work to diagnose conditions, develop new treatments, and contribute to evidence-based medicine. It allows them to form hypotheses and advance medical knowledge based on empirical evidence and clinical experience [1, 2].

B. Deductive inference (deduction is truth transferring and truth preserving, but not truth guaranteeing), in medicine involves making decisions based on established premises or information, following a logical process to reach a specific conclusion. This type of reasoning is commonly used in clinical diagnosis and treatment planning. Here's how deductive inference works in medicine:

Establishing Premises: Deductive inference starts with a set of established premises or facts. In medicine, these premises can be patient symptoms, medical history, diagnostic tests, and medical knowledge.

Identifying a Specific Case: When a patient presents with specific symptoms and clinical findings, these serve as the specific case under consideration.

Applying General Principles: The physician applies general medical principles, guidelines, and knowledge to the specific case. This involves using medical textbooks, guidelines, research findings, and clinical expertise.

Logical Reasoning: Deductive reasoning involves a step-by-step logical process. The healthcare provider uses known premises and general principles to make inferences about the specific case. This reasoning follows a structured path, with each step logically leading to the next.

Reaching a Conclusion: Based on the premises and logical reasoning, the physician reaches a specific conclusion regarding the patient's condition, diagnosis, or treatment plan.

Clinical Decision-Making: The conclusion derived from deductive inference guides clinical decision-making. It may involve prescribing a particular treatment, ordering further diagnostic tests, or deciding on a course of action.

Consideration of Uncertainty: It is important to acknowledge that deductive inference in medicine may not always lead to a definitive conclusion. Healthcare providers must also consider uncertainty and the possibility of differential diagnoses. They may use inductive reasoning, additional tests, or consultations to refine their conclusions.

Deductive inference is a vital aspect of medical decision-making, helping healthcare providers systematically assess and address patients' health issues. It allows for a structured approach to diagnosis and treatment, ensuring that medical decisions are based on sound logic and established medical knowledge. However, it is important to remember that medicine often involves complex and multifaceted cases, and deductive reasoning is just one part of the diagnostic process [1, 2].

C. Abductive Reasoning

It is a form of logical inference that involves making educated guesses or hypotheses to explain a set of observations or facts. It is commonly used when the available evidence is incomplete, uncertain, or lacks a straightforward explanation. In abductive reasoning, individuals seek the best possible explanation or hypothesis based on the information at hand. While it does not guarantee absolute truth, abductive reasoning is a valuable tool for generating plausible explanations in various fields, including science, medicine, law, and everyday problem-solving.

Here are the key characteristics of abductive reasoning:

1. Start with Observation: abductive reasoning begins with the observation of specific facts, data, or evidence. These observations may be incomplete or ambiguous.
2. Hypothesis Generation: Individuals generate one or more hypotheses or possible explanations that could account for the observed data. These hypotheses are typically based on patterns, associations, or prior knowledge.
3. Inference to the Best Explanation: The goal is to identify the hypothesis that offers the most plausible or best explanation for the observed evidence. This is not necessarily the only possible explanation but the one that seems most likely given the available information.
4. Testing and Verification: Once a hypothesis is proposed, it can be further tested, and new evidence can be collected to confirm or refute it. This may involve additional observations, experiments, or data collection.
5. Iterative Process: Abductive reasoning is often iterative, meaning that as new evidence or information becomes available, the hypothesis may need to be revised or refined.
6. Uncertainty and Probability: Abductive reasoning acknowledges uncertainty, and it assigns a degree of probability to each hypothesis. The hypothesis with the highest probability is considered the best explanation.
7. Open-Ended: Abductive reasoning is open-ended and does not always lead to a single definitive conclusion. It is used to explore and evaluate multiple possibilities.

Abductive reasoning is essential in scientific research, clinical diagnosis, problem-solving, and the formation of hypotheses in various disciplines. It allows individuals to make sense of complex or ambiguous situations by inferring likely explanations based on the available evidence. While it does not provide absolute certainty, it is a valuable cognitive process for generating understanding and insight when complete information is lacking [1, 2].

D. Probabilistic Reasoning.

Probabilistic reasoning is a fundamental concept in decision-making and inference that involves assessing and utilising probabilities to make informed choices, especially when dealing with uncertainty. It is a key component of fields like statistics, artificial intelligence, and various branches of science, including medicine and engineering. Here's a more detailed explanation of probabilistic reasoning:

1. Probabilities and Uncertainty: Probabilistic reasoning acknowledges that many real-world situations involve uncertainty. In these situations, it's often impossible to predict outcomes with certainty. Instead, probabilities are assigned to different possible outcomes based on available information and knowledge.
2. Bayesian Inference: Bayesian probability is a common framework for probabilistic reasoning. It is named after Thomas Bayes, an eighteenth-century statistician. In Bayesian inference, prior knowledge and new evidence are combined to update probabilities. This approach is widely used in various fields to make predictions and decisions.
3. Probabilistic Models: Probabilistic reasoning often involves creating and using probabilistic models. These models describe the relationships between variables, events, and outcomes. By incorporating probabilities into these models, it is possible to estimate the likelihood of specific events occurring.
4. Decision-Making: Probabilistic reasoning is essential in decision-making. When faced with multiple choices, decision-makers evaluate the probabilities associated with each choice and select the one that maximises expected value or utility. It is particularly useful when assessing risks and rewards in complex situations.
5. Statistical Inference: In statistics, probabilistic reasoning plays a crucial role in hypothesis testing and parameter estimation. Statistical tests provide p-values that indicate the likelihood of observing a particular result under a null hypothesis. Researchers use these probabilities to draw conclusions.
6. Decision Support Systems: Probabilistic reasoning is used in decision support systems to assist professionals in various fields, such as healthcare. These systems provide recommendations or suggestions based on available data and probabilities.
7. Risk Assessment: Probabilistic risk assessment is commonly used in fields like engineering, where it is important to evaluate the likelihood and consequences of various failures or accidents.

8. Diagnosis: In medicine, probabilistic reasoning is integral to clinical decision-making. Healthcare providers assess the likelihood of different medical conditions based on symptoms, test results, and risk factors. Bayesian networks are used to model complex relationships among variables in healthcare.
9. Uncertainty and Variability: Probabilistic reasoning acknowledges the inherent uncertainty and variability in medical practice. It helps healthcare professionals communicate the likelihood of different outcomes to patients, allowing them to make more informed decisions [1, 2].

In light of this and the fact that the knowledge base that we have is not absolute fact, unlike mathematics and logics, it means the decision we make is always a casualty of "fallibilism" [3].

Peirce's assertion that knowledge need not be exact raises concerns regarding the vagueness of the required justification. Peirce's fallibilism, which is a humble and adaptable approach to learning in light of the inherent limitations of our cognitive processes, methods, and tools.

1. Fallibilism, as an epistemological thesis, acknowledges the possibility of error in our beliefs, regardless of their strength or subject matter. As an epistemological recommendation, fallibilism encourages continuous learning and building upon our existing knowledge.
2. The process of acquiring knowledge requires a sense of humility, as we must accept that we could be wrong. Peirce's emphasis lies in ensuring that the path of genuine inquiry remains open and unobstructed.
3. Certainty and infallibility in claims to knowledge are elusive, given that our presumed sources of knowledge are susceptible to errors [4–7]. This is all to confirm that to be a human is to err.

References

1. Johansson I, Lynøe N. Medicine & philosophy. A twenty-first century introduction. Ontos Verlag. ISBN 978-3-938793-90-9. p. 1–5.
2. Beauchamp TL, Childress JF. Principles of biomedical ethics. Oxford: Oxford University Press; 1979.
3. Elizabeth F. COOKE, peirce, fallibilism, and the science of mathematics. Philos Math. 2003;11(2):158–75.
4. Peirce CS Collected Papers. C Hartshorne, P Weis, A W Burks (eds.). Cambridge: Harvard University Press, 1931–1958, (1. 13–14, c. 1897).
5. CS Pierce. The scientific attitude and Fallibilism." In Justus Buchler (ed.). Philosophical writings of Peirce. New York: Dover, 1955.
6. Pojman LP. What can we know? An introduction to the theory of knowledge. Belmont: Wadsworth; 2001.
7. Sorenson R. Vagueness. The Stanford encyclopedia of philosophy (Summer 2018 Edition), EN Zalta (ed) https://plato.stanford.edu/archives/sum/entries.

Chapter 18
Ethics and Decision-Making

The process of decision-making in medicine involves the following steps:

(1) Identify the problem. (2) Apply the local Code of Ethics. (3) Determine the nature of the dilemma. (4) Generate potential courses of action. (5) Consider the potential consequences of all options and determine a course of action. (6) Evaluate the selected course of action. (7) Seek a second opinion if not sure. (8) Implement the course of action [1, 2].

The Foundations

Healthcare professionals face ethical decision-making challenges in various settings, including clinical, educational, research, and home care. These decisions demand strict adherence to professional ethical standards and institutional ethical norms and legal requirements. Just like legal obligations, ignorance of ethical responsibilities is no excuse for non-compliance.

Numerous frameworks exist for ethical decision-making in healthcare. These models, governing patient care and health client services, are rooted in fundamental biomedical ethical principles of beneficence, non-maleficence, autonomy, and justice. They reflect essential professional attributes and responsibilities such as accountability, advocacy, altruism, autonomy (both for patients and professionals), compassion, competence, confidentiality, empathy, fidelity, fiduciary duty, loyalty, patience, social responsibility, teamwork, and truthfulness.

S. Abbas, *Medical Ethics*, https://doi.org/10.1007/978-981-96-9199-9_18

However, following these principles can be particularly challenging in the current managed care environment, which presents significant conflicts of interest. Most ethical decision-making models share core elements:

1. Identifying ethical problems, issues, or dilemmas.
2. Collecting pertinent facts and making reasonable assumptions.
3. Analysing various courses of action.
4. Selecting the best course of action based on ethical approaches, guidelines, and compliance with ethical and legal directives.

The systems approach enhances this model by introducing a feedback loop. Under this method, decision-makers continuously monitor and gather feedback on their chosen actions' appropriateness, efficacy, and effectiveness. If negative feedback suggests suboptimal performance, they modify their course of action accordingly. General systems theory serves as the basis for this approach.

Healthcare professionals are reminded that ignorance of their ethical responsibilities is not an excuse for non-compliance. Von Bertalanffy originally developed systems theory in the 1920s, and it is now widely used in engineering, natural sciences, and business and management.

Within the systems approach to ethical decision-making in healthcare, decision-makers must assess numerous relevant factors throughout the analysis, including:

1. Sociocultural considerations, such as gender, race, ethnicity, religion, and sexual orientation.
2. Legal implications tied to a decision.
3. Ethical requirements, ensuring alignment with professional codes of ethics or personal moral and ethical standards.
4. Economic impact on those affected by the decision.
5. Political consequences, if applicable.

In addition to considering these S-L-E-E-P factors, decision-makers should apply the principle of symmetry when resolving healthcare ethical issues. This principle involves a multidimensional analysis of a chosen course of action by assuming opposing perspectives and assessing implementation from each viewpoint [3] (Fig. 18.1).

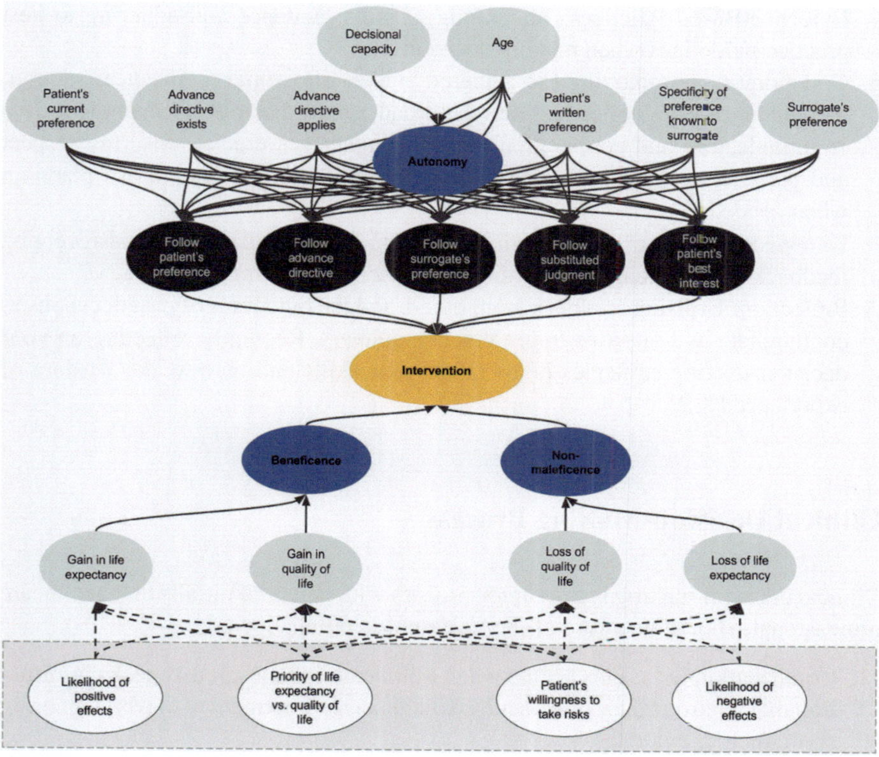

Fig. 18.1 Decision making process

Essential Clinical Skills

Effective clinical decision-making is the result of a harmonious blend of experience and various key skills, which encompass:

1. Pattern Recognition: Gaining insights from past experiences.
2. Critical Thinking: Employing an analytical, logical approach that separates decisions from emotions. This involves a certain level of skepticism, the ability to define objectives, examine assumptions, maintain an open mind, acknowledge personal biases, and evaluate supporting evidence.
3. Communication Skills: Active listening plays a pivotal role in understanding the patient's story, unearthing what remains unsaid, their experiences, and their desires. This paves the way for a patient-centric approach that encourages self-management. Furthermore, effective information delivery is vital to ensure that patients, clients, their caregivers, and family members are actively engaged in the decision-making process, comprehending the information provided.

4. Evidence-Based Practices: Integrating existing evidence and adhering to best practice guidelines when making decisions.
5. Collaboration: Employing the gathered evidence to solicit assistance, support, and guidance from colleagues and the broader multidisciplinary team. Effective communication and cooperation with colleagues are crucial, ensuring respect and persistence when seeking support, thus facilitating collaborative planning when needed.
6. Knowledge Sharing: Actively sharing your learning experiences and receiving feedback from colleagues regarding your decision-making processes.
7. Reflection: Utilising feedback from others and the outcomes of past decisions to contemplate and improve future practice delivery. Regularly reflecting on your decision-making strategies helps refine your skills and harness the wisdom of experience [1, 2].

Clinical Decision-Making Process

Clinical decision-making is a complex process with potential pitfalls that healthcare professionals should be aware of. Some common pitfalls include:

1. Confirmation Bias: This occurs when a clinician subconsciously seeks information that confirms their preconceived diagnosis or treatment plan while ignoring contradictory evidence.
2. Availability Bias: Clinicians may be influenced by recent cases or vivid experiences, leading them to overemphasise the importance of these cases in their decision-making, even when they are not representative of typical cases.
3. Anchoring Bias: This happens when a clinician relies too heavily on the first piece of information they receive (the "anchor") and doesn't adjust their thinking as new information becomes available.
4. Overconfidence: Clinicians may overestimate their own knowledge and abilities, leading to unwarranted certainty in their decisions.
5. Diagnostic Momentum: This occurs when a diagnosis is made early in the clinical encounter, and subsequent information is interpreted in a way that confirms the initial diagnosis, even if it might not be correct.
6. Ignoring Patient Preferences: Failing to involve patients in the decision-making process or ignoring their values and preferences can lead to suboptimal outcomes.
7. Communication: Inadequate communication and collaboration among healthcare team members can lead to misunderstandings and poor decision-making.
8. Fatigue and Stress: Healthcare professionals working long hours under high levels of stress or fatigue may experience impaired judgment and decision-making abilities.
9. Lack of Time: Time constraints in clinical settings can lead to rushed decisions and missed opportunities for thorough evaluation.

10. Cognitive Load: Overwhelming clinicians with excessive information can lead to information overload and poor decision-making.
11. Diagnostic Momentum: This occurs when a diagnosis is made early in the clinical encounter, and subsequent information is interpreted in a way that confirms the initial diagnosis, even if it might not be correct [4, 5].

In medicine, heuristics are commonly used to solve problems quickly. These informal problem-solving techniques help experts arrive at solutions quickly, drawing from their experience. However, healthcare professionals must recognize that while heuristics are essential for making decisions in a high-pressure environment, they should be subject to regular assessment and integrated into a structured problem-solving framework to enhance consistency and precision in clinical judgments.

To optimise our decision-making process, we must amalgamate our knowledge, expertise, and past mistakes. We must be vigilant during stressful or fatigued states to prevent simplistic decision-making models.

1. Pattern Recognition: Many of us were trained to recognise patterns in medical school. When we encounter a young person with chest pain, we often think of anxiety or musculoskeletal issues.
2. Scientific Method: Each patient interaction can be viewed as a research project, where we define a problem, formulate hypotheses, collect and analyse data, and confirm or reject our hypotheses.
3. Probabilities: Evaluating probabilities is integral to our decision-making process. This involves assessing the likelihood of a particular outcome based on available data.
4. Differential Diagnoses: we generate differential diagnosis lists, time constraints and practicality often lead us to shorten the list. However, we should remain vigilant for the rare cases.
5. Tests: Test results significantly impact clinical decisions. It's important to understand the limitations of the tests, which are not definitive.
6. Treatment Thresholds: Deciding on a treatment often involves establishing thresholds that must be met before initiating a specific treatment. The threshold varies depending on the potential benefits and risks of treatment. For example, treatments with substantial benefits and low risks have a lower threshold, while those with limited benefits and moderate risks require a higher threshold. This threshold concept guides our treatment decisions, considering the trade-offs between potential benefits and risks.

In complex cases, treatment decisions can be challenging, particularly when the treatment is invasive and has a significant risk for complications [5, 6].

The estimate that 44,000–98,000 patients die each year in the United States due to medical errors is alarming, shedding light on critical healthcare issues. These errors, distinct from underlying medical conditions, occur at various stages of patient care, from diagnosis to treatment, involving factors like misdiagnoses, medication errors, and communication breakdowns. The consequences extend beyond patients to their families, underscoring the urgent need for quality improvements, standardised procedures, and patient advocacy. To address this global concern, research, regulatory measures, and a culture of safety and transparency are essential. In conclusion, these statistics emphasise the imperative of enhancing patient safety and require collaboration among healthcare providers, policymakers, and the public to prevent such avoidable tragedies [7].

Practical Wisdom in Decision-Making

Clinical diagnosis shares similarities with detective work rather than pure scientific inquiry. A closer examination of the diagnostic process reveals the following stages:

1. Collecting Information: Patients interpret symptoms through their own frame of reference, making it essential to avoid leading questions. As data is recounted, it can unintentionally change. Being vigilant during patient examination is crucial; we must observe carefully and avoid missing key findings.
2. Formulating Hypotheses: We employ many strategies to create a list of differential diagnoses, adapting them based on our knowledge and the patient's condition.
3. Testing Hypotheses: This process involves evaluating potential solutions to determine the most likely or accurate one. Physicians and healthcare providers use a combination of clinical knowledge, diagnostic tests, and patient assessments to test these hypotheses and arrive at a final diagnosis or treatment plan.
4. Rule Out Worst Case Scenarios.
   This strategy prioritises risk assessment but may sometimes leave our primary diagnostic inquiry unresolved. For instance, when dealing with acute chest pain, we might rule out numerous severe conditions without arriving at a definitive diagnosis.
5. Reflecting on Findings: Reflection in clinical practice is essential for healthcare providers. It improves Quality: Identifies areas for clinical practice enhancement, leverages Experience, enables learning from past decisions for better future choices, prioritises Patients, considers patient perspectives and promotes patient-centred care, assesses Ethics: Evaluates alignment with ethical standards, fosters Development: Supports ongoing professional growth and knowledge updates, reduces errors and identifies past errors to prevent future ones [8].

Once we have gathered the pertinent case information, how can we ensure the integrity of our thought processes? It is crucial to have insight into the issues and practice metacognition, meaning being conscious of how we think. As we make decisions, we should reflect on the decision-making process, being vigilant about biases and hasty errors. We can evolve our clinical reasoning from unconscious reactions to that of accomplished thinkers. Employing cognitive forcing techniques, like structured data review and diagnostic checklists, is beneficial. Reducing reliance on memory through resources is essential. Being accountable to our team for our thought processes, even "thinking out loud" during ward rounds, encourages scrutiny when our reasoning is flawed. Training tools like the One Minute Preceptor can help trainees develop thinking skills and keep us sharp as supervisors. Equally important is honing error recognition and recovery skills.

Then we ask ourselves: what is the best solution for this patient? In this regard, the thinking doctor should also be a considerate doctor. We have to address the holistic patient's needs, displaying kindness and genuine interest in their humanity, a quality essential for effective patient care.

Edmund Pellegrino emphasises the essence of the clinical encounter in medicine, encapsulated in three key questions:

Identifying the Problem: The clinical encounter begins with diagnosis, where physicians assess patients' symptoms and complaints to identify health issues.

Exploring Solutions: Healthcare providers, drawing from their expertise, consider various treatment options and evaluate their pros and cons.

Personalising Care: The final step involves tailoring a patient-centred solution, considering the individual's unique needs, values, and medical history.

Pellegrino's approach underscores patient-centred care, ethics, and the art and science of medicine. It's about asking the right questions and making empathetic, well-informed decisions in patient care [9, 10].

Practical Wisdom in Ethical Decision

In medical decision-making, physicians must exhibit wisdom due to the complexity of illness and the ever-evolving landscape of biomedical science and therapeutic options. Wisdom is viewed through two primary accounts: virtuous character traits within the physician and thoughtful consideration of care goals and decision-making elements. In medicine, wisdom is linked to ethics, which promote the well-being of patients, including health, dignity, and autonomy. Promoting this well-being requires respectful dialogue focused on the patient's best interests. Medicine is a moral practice requiring a holistic understanding of science and ethics. This enables physicians to treat patients not just as bodies afflicted with diseases, but as individuals facing health challenges [11].

Shared decision-making (SDM) has been promoted as a collaborative approach between clinicians and patients. Proponents argue that patients have a right to be actively involved in decisions concerning their health and well-being, while others emphasise the utilitarian benefits, such as improved adherence to management plans and better health outcomes, associated with greater patient involvement.

It is widely agreed that true shared decision-making can only occur when both the doctor and patient commit to the collaborative decision-making process. In pursuit of this goal, efforts have been made to identify the competencies required for SDM in clinical practice and to teach and assess these competencies among medical students, trainee doctors, and senior clinicians.

While many studies have explored patient preferences for various decision-making styles and the extent to which these preferences are met, there's a notable absence of research on clinicians' preferences and experiences with different clinical decision-making approaches.

Various factors contribute to this situation, including structural constraints, perceived time limitations during consultations, and a lack of comprehensive information that would enable patients to meaningfully participate in the decision-making process. Moreover, the inherent power dynamics in the doctor–patient relationship mean that physician preferences and behaviours are likely to influence patients' ability to engage in the decision-making process [12–15].

The health and well-being of individuals depend on medical and public health decision-making processes. There is a call for the incorporation of phronesis, or practical wisdom, in medical-related ethical decision-making as a complement to evidence-based practice.

Some have argued that doctors follow deontological (rule-based) approaches to medical decision-making, but the overwhelming quantity of these guidelines makes it increasingly unmanageable. Estimates suggest that there are more than 7000 deontological guidelines for clinicians to follow, with new ones added regularly. The rigid nature of these principles fails to account for the complexities of caring for patients with multiple comorbidities and in challenging circumstances.

Doctors are vulnerable because they must meet growing patient, colleague, and society expectations while balancing limited resources and healthcare priorities. Our theory aims to make ethical decision-making more manageable, reducing feelings of vulnerability, and building physician resilience.

Phronesis, in this context, represents accumulated wisdom derived from previous practice dilemmas and decisions. It is an "executive virtue" that prioritises the involvement of stakeholders in the decision-making process, enabling ethical choices to be effectively implemented. One problem in clinical settings is uncertainty, particularly about diagnostic accuracy and the effectiveness of treatments. Understanding and respecting patients' preferences and other stakeholders' needs are also important. When multiple moral and social factors intersect, medical decision-makers may be unsure about what is best for patients and society, as well as how to achieve optimal outcomes for both. Toulmin and MacIntyre advocate for the recovery of practical Phronesis, like Aristotle's phronesis, as a judgment to resolve conflicts and disagreements. Without moral virtues, phronesis can guide the right means to achieve genuine moral ends. Both moral virtues and phronesis are essential for ethical decision-making [16–18].

Virtue (V.)	POLE1(excess)	Mean	POLE2 (deficiency)
1	Doctor decides	Negotiation	Patient decides
2	ALL get treatment	Justice/fairness	Select few get treated
3	Overly trusted	Trustworthiness/(including maintaining confidentiality)	No trust
4	Constant litigation worry	Lawfulness	Ignore legal constraints
5	Constantly seeks guidance from peers and/or professional bodies	Collaboration (making collaborative decisions/seek guidance)	Self –guided/does not consult
6	Use own values and beliefs	Cultural competence	Go with patient's values and beliefs only
7	Too involved (over emotional)	Emotional intelligence (including interpersonal communication)	Distant/aloof
8	Treat at all cost	Awareness of limits to treatments	Limited consideration of treatment options
9	Constant mentoring/overly directive	Mentorship (and being an approachable mentor)	No interest in mentorship
10	Trying to cater to all aspects—Arts/humanities science, spiritual and physical	Balanced approach	Just one approach—e.g. science/clinical only
11	Over-analytical (navel gazing)	Reflexive	Never reflect
12	Foolhardy risk taker	Courage (to speak out and act)	Cowardice (avoids conflict)
13	Thinking they are bullet proof	Resilience	Avoidance of any stress
14	Obsessed with finances/ resources	Resource awareness	No consideration of resources
15	Seen it all/know it all/can deal with anything	Phronesis	

Conroy et al.: This table represents the consolidated 'collective practical wisdom' conveyed in the decision narratives.

The table above displays a continuum of virtues, including phronesis, and the range of actions associated with each virtue, spanning from deficiency to excess, with a midpoint. This table illustrates the amalgamated "collective practical wisdom" derived from the decision narratives shared by the participants in the study Hence, they posit that it is feasible to nurture phronesis by means of introspection and discussion, fostering the capacity to make decisions that align with the unique circumstances and contexts encountered by practitioners [18].

These virtues collectively reflect the "collective practical wisdom" distilled from the decision narratives provided by medical practitioners, capturing the diversity of perspectives and experiences within the medical community It is important to note that these virtues are not an exhaustive list to be universally followed but rather serve as a catalyst for reflection, nurturing phronesis through reflection and debate to facilitate sound decision-making across a range of cases and contexts.

This approach aligns with the theory that consensus on virtues among a group of practitioners fosters sound practice. The flexibility of this continuum allows practitioners to merge or incorporate virtues according to their preferences, promoting diversity within the community and enhancing practical wisdom. This concept extends to community-based moral reasoning, emphasising the role of medical knowledge and virtues in shaping ethically wise decisions. Seeking guidance from colleagues with experiential knowledge is crucial in complex scenarios, while resource constraints and concerns about litigation also influence decision-making. These tensions can be resolved through moral discourse and the application of this resource [9, 16, 18, 19, 20].

We need to direct resources to facilitate the practice of virtue ethics/phronesis-based ethical decision-making in the medical field. While some critics argue that this approach is challenging to attain and that phronesis takes various forms, our conceptualisation aligns with the practice virtue ethics version. Given the evolving role of doctors from sole knowledge guardians to facilitators of wise decisions, this approach holds both conceptual and practical relevance.

These virtues offer practical wisdom for moral debates related to ethical decision-making in professional education and practice. This approach contributes to professional fulfilment and excellence by fostering moral reasoning, making it integral to diagnosis, care planning, and the best interests of patients and the community.

The intellectual virtue of phronesis guides practitioners on where to act along the continuum, ensuring that moral reasoning and relevance go hand in hand. It also enriches the teaching of ethics, particularly for medical students by consolidating the fifteen virtue continua as "Collective Practical Wisdom."

Rather than offering a deontological prescription, it provides a stimulus for reflection in both undergraduate and postgraduate medical education and continuous professional development programs [11, 18, 19].

In addition to augmenting the expertise of experienced professionals, medical trainees need not postpone their journey to wisdom or make wise decisions until they gain more experience. Rather, they can begin learning elements of phronesis from the broader medical community early in their careers. Future developments in medical decision-making, research, and policy stand to gain significant advantages by embracing this non-prescriptive approach, ultimately enhancing the health and well-being of patients and society at large and combating codification of medicine that and promote personalised medicine. There is an understanding that "the aim of medical education is to develop doctors who are reflective, empathetic, trustworthy, committed to patient welfare and able to deal with complexity and uncertainty" [20].

References

1. Beauchamp TL, Childress JF. Principles of biomedical ethics. 7th ed. New York: Oxford University Press; 2012.
2. Bradley LJ, Hendricks CB. Ethical decision making: basic issues. Fam J. 2008;16:261–3.
3. Scott R. Chapter 2 - Ethical foundations. In: Promoting legal and ethical awareness. Mosby; 2009. p. 24–49.
4. Groopman J. How doctors think. Boston: Houghton Mifflin; 2007.
5. Borrell-Carrio F, Epstein RM. Preventing errors in clinical practice: a call for self-awareness. Ann Fam Med. 2004;2:310–6.
6. Woolever DR. The art and science of clinical decision making. Fam Pract Manag. 2008 May;15(5):31–6.
7. Kohn L, Corrigan J, Donaldson M, editors. To err is human: building a safer health system. Washington, DC: National Academy Press; 2000.
8. Croskerry P. Achieving quality in clinical decision making: cognitive strategies and detection of bias. Acad Emerg Med. 2002;9:1184–204.
9. Pellegrino E. Thomasma D. A philosophical basis of medical practice: towards a philosophy and ethic of the healing professions. Oxford: Oxford University Press; 1980.
10. Dror I. A novel approach to minimize error in the medical domain: cognitive neuroscientific insights into training. Med Teach. 2011;33:34–8.
11. Kaldjian L. Wisdom in medical decision-making. In: Sternberg R, Glück J, editors. The Cambridge handbook of wisdom (Cambridge handbooks in psychology). Cambridge: Cambridge University Press; 2019. p. 698–720.
12. Murray E, Pollack L, White M, et al. Clinical decision-making: physicians' preferences and experiences. BMC Fam Pract. 2007;8:10.
13. Stevenson FA. General practitioners' views on shared decision making: a qualitative analysis. Patient Educ Couns. 2003;50:291–3. https://doi.org/10.1016/S0738-3991(03)00052-1.
14. Charles C, Gafni A, Whelan T. Self-reported use of shared decision-making among breast cancer specialists and perceived barriers and facilitators to implementing this approach. Health Expect. 2004;7:338–48.
15. Wills CE, Holmes-Rovner M. Patient comprehension of information for shared treatment decision making: state of the art and future directions. Patient Educ Couns. 2003;50:285–90.
16. MacIntyre A, After virtue. A study in moral theory. London: Gerald Duckworth & Co. Ltd; 1981.
17. Toulmin S. How medicine saved the life of ethics. Perspect Biol Med. 1982;25(4):736–50.
18. Conroy M, Malik AY, Hale C, et al. Using practical wisdom to facilitate ethical decision-making: a major empirical study of *phronesis* in the decision narratives of doctors. BMC Med Ethics. 2021;22:16.
19. Oakley J. Virtue theory. In: Ashcroft R, Dawson A, Draper H, McMillan J, editors. Principles of healthcare ethics. Wiley; 2007. p. 87–91.
20. Campbell AV, Chin J, Voo TC. How can we know that ethics education produces ethical doctors? Med Teach. 2007;29(5):431–6.

Chapter 19
Shared Decision Making

SDM involves providing individuals with support to:

Comprehend the available care, treatment, and support options, as well as the associated risks, benefits, and consequences.

Make an informed decision regarding their preferred course of action, guided by evidence-based, high-quality information, and their personal preferences. Therefore, SDM is a collaborative process where clinicians and individuals work together to choose tests, treatments, management, or support options. These decisions are grounded in both evidence and the individual's well-informed preferences that include doing nothing.

Shared decision-making (SDM), a shift away from clinicians making unilateral decisions for patients, is gaining momentum in healthcare policy. Fundamentally, SDM is based on the idea that individual self-determination is a valuable objective, and it is the responsibility of clinicians to assist patients in reaching this goal whenever possible. SDM involves clinicians and patients sharing the best available evidence when faced with decisions, with the goal of supporting patients in considering their options and achieving informed preferences. While its earliest mention dates back to 1982, the concept builds upon the principles of patient-centred care. Nevertheless, despite attention to these principles and competencies, there remains a lack of clear guidance on how to implement SDM in regular practice to facilitate personalised care. Personalised care is put into practice through the Comprehensive Model for Personalised Care. Developed collaboratively with diverse stakeholders, this model integrates six evidence-based and interconnected components, each characterised by a standardised, reproducible delivery framework. These components consist of:

- Shared decision-making
- Personalised care
- Empowering choice, encompassing legal entitlements
- Social prescribing and community-based support
- Supported self-management

S. Abbas, *Medical Ethics*, https://doi.org/10.1007/978-981-96-9199-9_19

- Personal health budgets.

Shared decision-making has gained support as a way to involve patients in their healthcare choices, driven by beliefs in patient rights and autonomy and the practical benefits of enhancing adherence and health outcomes. Regardless of the motivation, it is agreed that successful shared decision-making requires commitment from both doctors and patients. To promote this, efforts have been made to define the competencies required for shared decision-making in clinical settings, as well as to educate and evaluate these skills in medical trainees and practicing physicians.

Charles et al. conducted a survey of breast cancer specialists in Ontario to gauge the degree to which they practiced shared decision-making, their comfort with the approach, and their perceived challenges and facilitators in implementing it [1].

Nationally representative data on physicians' perspectives are essential to inform interventions aimed at promoting shared decision-making. Many patients are not experiencing the level of involvement they desire in clinical decision-making. This discrepancy can be attributed to various factors, including structural limitations, perceived time constraints during consultations, and insufficient or inadequate information provided to patients, hindering their meaningful participation in the decision-making process [2, 3]. Given the greater influence physicians often have in the doctor–patient relationship, it is likely that their preferences and actions impact patients' ability to engage in the decision-making process. Currently, it was estimated that 73% of doctors make shared decisions with patients, 15% make decisions based on paternalism (mostly older doctors and doctors trained in non-western institutions) and 12% prefer that patients and their families to make the decision (consumerism) [4, 5].

SDM acknowledges the importance of fostering autonomy by establishing positive relationships and showing respect for individual competence and reliance on others. It was first described in 1982 "The ethical foundation of informed consent can be traced to the promotion of two values: personal well-being and self-determination. To ensure that these values are respected and enhanced, the Commission finds that patients… must have all relevant information regarding their condition and alternative treatments, including possible benefits, risks, costs, other consequences, and significant uncertainties.… Ethically valid consent is a process of shared decision making based upon mutual respect and participation" [5].

These principles are central to both self-determination and relational autonomy. Self-determination theory focuses on our natural inclinations to safeguard and enhance our well-being. Relational autonomy refers to the perspective that while we have some degree of autonomy, our choices are invariably linked to interpersonal relationships and mutual dependencies and honouring informed preferences, the initial step for proponents of implementing SDM is to secure support for the underlying rationale from clinicians and other stakeholders [6, 7].

Before proceeding, it is important to acknowledge the challenges clinicians may face. Barriers to SDM include low health literacy and patients from cultural backgrounds with less emphasis on individual decision-making. Hence, it is crucial to emphasise that SDM must be rooted in strong clinical communication skills. This includes the development of rapport and structuring effective consultations [8]. SDM is backed by findings from 86 randomised trials, demonstrating increased patient knowledge, enhanced decision confidence, greater patient engagement, and, often, a preference for more conservative treatment options among informed patients. Resulting in decisions that are better comprehended, grounded in more precise expectations regarding potential outcomes, and aligned with individual preferences [9].

The Process

Elwyn et al. suggested a three steps process

Choice Talk: Initiating the Decision-Making Process

Choice talk involves informing patients that reasonable options exist and can be carried out through various means, not solely in face-to-face conversations. For example, a patient with hyperthyroidism might be advised to use a decision support website.

Components of choice talk include: (a) Step back: Begin by summarising the situation, saying, "Now that we have identified the problem, it's time to think about what to do next." (b) Offer choice: Patients may sometimes misinterpret the presentation of options. To prevent this, explain, "There is valuable information about how these treatments differ that I'd like to discuss with you." (c) Justify choice: Emphasise the importance of respecting individual preferences and the role of uncertainty.

Personalising Preferences: Clarify that different issues hold varying significance for different people, e.g., "Treatments have different consequences, and some will matter more to you than to others."

Uncertainty: Many patients are unaware of the extent of uncertainty in medicine. Highlight that treatments are not always effective, and individual outcomes can be unpredictable, e.g., "Treatments are not always effective, and the chances of experiencing side effects vary." (d) Check Reaction: Given the array of options, some patients may feel unsettled. Use phrases like "Shall we go on?" or "Shall I tell you about the options?" (e) Defer Closure: If some patients ask clinicians to "tell me what to do," it's advisable to postpone closure, assuring your willingness to support the process. For instance, say, "I'm happy to share my views and help you make a good decision. But before I do so, may I describe the options in more detail so that you understand what is at stake?."

Options Talk: Detailing the Available Choices

(a) Check Knowledge: Patients, even well-informed ones, may lack awareness of options, associated benefits, and drawbacks. Inquire, "What have you heard or read about the treatment of prostate cancer?" (b) List Options: Create a clear list of the available choices, providing a structured framework. Write them down and say, "Let me list the options before we delve into more details." If applicable, include "watchful waiting" or use positive terms like "active surveillance." (c) Describe Options: Encourage dialogue and explore preferences. Explain the options in practical terms. For instance, if there are two medical treatments, say, "Both options are similar and involve taking medication regularly." Highlight any significant differences (e.g., surgery or medication), where postponement is possible, or when decisions are reversible. Say, "These options will have different implications for you compared to other people, so I want to describe…"

Harms and Benefits: Clearly presenting the pros and cons of each option is central to shared decision-making. Learn about effective risk communication, framing effects, and the importance of providing risk data in both absolute and relative terms. Consider presenting information in "chunks." (d) Provide Patient Decision Support: Tools that make options visible and save time can be beneficial. Some are concise enough for use in clinical encounters. Examples include Issues Cards, Decision Boards, and Option Grids. Shared decision making may require more than one encounter, and more extensive patient decision-support tools may play a crucial role. Say, "These tools are designed to help you understand options in more detail. Use them, and return with any questions." (e) Summarise: Reiterate the options and assess understanding by asking for rephrased explanations, employing a "teach-back" method to check for misconceptions.

Decision Talk: Guiding Towards a Decision

(a) Focus on Preferences: Help the patient form preferences. Suggested phrases include, "What, from your point of view, matters most to you?" (b) Elicit a Preference: Be ready with a backup plan by offering more time or guidance if the patient wishes. (c) Moving to a Decision: Assess the need to either postpone or make a decision. Use phrases such as "Are you ready to decide?" or "Do you want more time? Do you have more questions?" and ask if there are more topics to discuss. (d) Offer Review: Remind the patient, when feasible, that decisions can be reviewed as a way to reach closure [10]. This model represents an evolution of prior work in this field, synthesising various contributions. It recognises its ethical foundations and the stages and skills outlined in previous research. However, the impetus for this three-step model emerged from our experiences in implementation studies. The primary objective is to assist clinicians in seamlessly incorporating shared decision-making (SDM) and patient decision support into their practice.

Many clinicians may initially resist the idea of adding further tasks to their clinical encounters. We acknowledge this concern and maintain that new systems must be established to adequately incentivise patient-centred care. Implementing brief decision support interventions can serve as a catalyst for a renewed dialogue and can facilitate the practical integration of SDM into busy clinical settings. This may require multiple encounters for some patients to discuss significant decisions [10].

Shared Decision Making (SDM) is a healthcare approach that places a strong emphasis on collaboration and active participation by both healthcare providers and patients. In this process, clinicians and patients come together to make informed choices regarding various aspects of healthcare, such as diagnostic tests, treatment plans, management strategies, and support options. Here is a more detailed elaboration of this statement:

1. Collaborative Process: SDM is characterised by healthcare providers and patients' active involvement in decision-making. It is a departure from the traditional model where clinicians make decisions on patients' behalf.
2. Choosing Tests and Treatments: SDM can include selecting the best diagnostic tests to identify a medical condition and deciding on the best treatment options.
3. Management and Support Options: SDM extends to patients and clinicians choosing the most suitable management strategies, such as rehabilitation plans, monitoring of chronic conditions, or long-term care options.
4. Grounded in Evidence: In SDM, healthcare providers discuss the risks, benefits, and potential consequences of each option with patients and provide them with the best available medical knowledge.
5. Informed Preferences: SDM recognises the importance of individual patient preferences. Healthcare choices are deeply personal, and what might be the best course of action for one patient may not be the same for another [11].

Healthcare systems need to empower people by listening to their informed preferences. By consolidating the choices of informed individuals on a broader scale, we can design and deliver services that match their preferences. This approach allows for more efficient allocation of resources.

References

1. Charles C, Gafni A, Whelan T. Self-reported use of shared decision-making among breast cancer specialists and perceived barriers and facilitators to implementing this approach. Health Expect. 2004;7:338.
2. Godolphin W, Towle A, McKendry R. Evaluation of the quality of patient information to support informed shared decision-making. Health Expect. 2001;4:235.
3. Wills CE, Holmes-Rovner M. Patient comprehension of information for shared treatment decision making: state of the art and future directions. Patient Educ Couns. 2003;50:285–90.
4. Murray E, Pollack L, White M, et al. Clinical decision-making: physicians' preferences and experiences. BMC Fam Pract. 2007;8:10. https://doi.org/10.1186/1471-2296-8-10.

5. President's Commission for the Study of Ethical Problems in Medicine and Biomedical and Behavioral Research. Making Health Care Decisions. The ethical and legal implications of informed consent in the patient–practitioner relationship. Washington, DC; 1982.
6. Ryan R, Deci E. Self-determination theory and the facilitation of intrinsic motivation, social development, and well-being. Am Psychol. 2000;55(1):68–78.
7. Mackenzie C. Relational autonomy, normative authority and perfectionism. J Soc Philos. 2008;39(4):512–33.
8. Braddock CH, Fihn SD, Levinson W, Jonsen AR, Pearlman RA. How doctors and patients discuss routine clinical decisions: informed decision making in the outpatient setting. J Gen Intern Med. 1997;12:339–45.
9. Stacey D, Bennett C, Barry M, Col N, Eden K, Holmes-Rovner M, Llewellyn-Thomas H, Lyddiatt A, et al. Decision aids for people facing health treatment or screening decisions. Cochrane Database Syst Rev. 2001.
10. Elwyn G, Frosch D, Thomson R, Joseph-Williams N, Lloyd A, Kinnersley P, Cording E, Tomson D, Dodd C, Rollnick S, Edwards A, Barry M. Shared decision making: a model for clinical practice. J Gen Intern Med. 2012;27(10):1361–7.
11. https://www.gmc-uk.org/ethical-guidance/ethical-guidance-for-doctors/good-medical-practice

Chapter 20
Medicine and the Humanities

Until the twentieth century, the theoretical demarcation line in the study of living processes resided in the debate between *physicalism and vitalism.* Physicalists claimed there was no fundamental difference between living organisms and inanimate matter. Living phenomena could therefore be studied and explained with the methods and laws of physics. This approach was strongly opposed by vitalists, who postulated that living organisms had properties that could not be reduced to physics or chemistry and, therefore, biological phenomena could not be analysed with the concepts or methods of those sciences. The advancement of cellular and evolutionary theories showed that traditional explanations for living processes, like Newtonian physics or non-material life forces, were inadequate. To resolve this challenge, a new concept emerged: organicism. Organicism explains life processes by relying on physiochemical and evolutionary concepts [1].

In clinical medicine, it is clear that using only biological information isn't enough to understand people's diverse experiences. As the medical community moved away from ideas that focus on the body or the physical world, a new theoretical boundary was established.

Reductionism and Holism

Reductionism and holism in medicine are now different. In medicine, the reductionist approach seeks to understand human illnesses using biological principles. Holists have tried to integrate social, cultural, and personal factors into medical theory. This division grew more pronounced in the latter part of the 20th century due to rapid advancements in molecular biology, genetics, and increasingly sophisticated medical technology [2].

Since the 1960s, a critical social movement has challenged the dominance of science and technology. This influence extended to medical schools. Medical education, they argued, had been neglecting critical aspects of medical practice, such as

S. Abbas, *Medical Ethics*, https://doi.org/10.1007/978-981-96-9199-9_20

the individual patient's experience of their illness and the societal factors, including poverty and social deprivation. Instead Students were taught to adopt "the medical gaze," which encouraged them to perceive individuals as culturally constructed entities identified primarily as cases or patients. This approach tended to disregard the significance of a person's unique experiences and cultural context [3].

To address these concerns, many medical faculties in the United States introduced courses on social sciences and humanities to their curricula. The goal was to bridge the gap between scientific knowledge and human experience, aiming to cultivate more compassionate physicians and restore medicine's status as a learned profession. This trend, often referred to as "Medical Humanities," has become a significant part of medical education in the U.S. and is gaining traction in European faculties.

While the holistic approach in medicine has revealed limitations in reductionist approaches to understanding human illness and highlighted various complex human phenomena in medical practice, it has not yet yielded a robust conceptual framework for advancing our comprehension of medicine. As Cassell laments, "it is one thing to emphasise wholeness, but quite another to develop the intellectual tools to address them. The holistic medicine movement serves as a cautionary example of what can occur when new concerns emerge without the accompanying development of new understanding or tools to manage them." [4]

Biopsychosocial Model

The biopsychosocial model is based on general systems theory. This model says that reality is made up of a hierarchy. The biological part is the same, but the other parts are different. These different parts come from scientific disciplines, like biology, chemistry, and physics. The doctor mixes these different approaches to address the patient's needs. This is Engel's concept of medicine, where the physician takes on the role of a "participant observer." As they attend to the patient's concerns, they utilise their personal inner perspective to compare and clarify the information. This approach emphasises the patient as an active initiator and collaborator rather than a mere object of study. The fundamental methodological triad for clinical investigation encompasses observation (external perspective), introspection (internal perspective), and dialogue (interviews), ultimately transforming the patient's data into scientific insights "The physician as scientist operates concurrently in two modes, one observational, the other relational." [5]

The clinical approach should prioritise the well-being of the patient, whether they are unwell or in good health, while still enabling the physician to maintain their scientific reasoning and actions. Pellegrino and Thomasma say that medicine is more than biology, physics, chemistry, or psychology. They see it as a relationship between two people where one seeks out the other to help with healing. They say that this interaction, and the nature of the relationship, is what makes medicine special [6].

These approaches all try to expand medical theory beyond its biological foundation. They emphasise the central role of medical consultation in this process, advocating for the inclusion of humanities and social sciences in medical theory and education. Humanities are seen as a means for physicians to enhance their comprehension of the human condition, as well as the individual qualities and distinctiveness of each patient. Social sciences, on the other hand, address the broader context within which the healing process occurs. However, in these approaches, humanities often appear as a supplemental component to medicine's biological knowledge base. Their primary function seems to be educational, aimed at promoting more humane behaviour among doctors, or in the words of Cassell, transforming medicine into a "learned profession." [4]

here are still questions, but we think activity theory could help us understand medical practice. Activity theory is a way of thinking that comes from the cultural–historical school of psychology. It developed during the 1920s when Lev Vygotsky and his associates studied how people learn and use language. Leontiev developed activity theory after Vygotsky. It explains how people act as a result of their environment. It is also important because it explains how expertise is gained. In modern technological settings, activity theory has interesting applications. Medical progress is the knowledge of human health and sickness, with the linguistic and technological instruments used in medical diagnosis and therapy. Over the history of interactions between physicians and their patients, medical notions have evolved. These notions are reflections of the medical field within the framework of actual practice. They contribute to the comprehension of a patient's condition as an integral aspect of the practice.

Both the patient and the physician use concepts to form a diagnosis based on the patient's symptoms and the signs detected by the physician. This diagnosis guides the physician's reflective analysis and responses to the patient's concerns [7].

Various medical specialties have unique toolsets and methods for constructing their diagnostic and therapeutic approaches, shaped by historical and cultural factors. Verbal communication, although common to all, is integrated with specialised tools. Physicians also use verbalisations for patient guidance, reassurance, and comfort and the therapeutic environment itself can be considered a tool domain.

Surgeons focus on physical issues like hernias and bowel obstruction while psychiatrists prioritise mental health concerns in patients with physical conditions. Consequently, the structure of the physician–patient relationship varies based on perceived focus [8].

Culture

The humanities play a crucial role in understanding the cultural and historical dimensions of medicine, challenging the assumption of universality in medical concepts, and highlighting the importance of considering the patient's unique cultural context. Medicine's central features include sign-mediated interactions, cultural contextuality, and the historical development of medical concepts. Clinical knowledge, according to Toulmin, is fundamentally historical, as it seeks to trace the sequence of events that led the patient to seek medical help. Moreover, when examining the patient's body from a biological perspective, it is considered a dynamic entity, constantly changing over time. Therefore, taking the patient's medical history is essential for understanding the body's natural history.

Clinical knowledge is also culturally influenced, requiring a shared understanding between the physician and patient regarding symptoms, behaviour interpretation, and ailment causation. This becomes particularly crucial when the patient comes from a different cultural background. Psychiatric concepts can vary significantly across cultures, leading to misunderstandings and misdiagnoses. It is important to interpret a patient's life history within their cultural context to avoid such pitfalls.

This suggests that the assumption that psychiatric concepts implying values and ideals are universally applicable needs to be questioned. The first step to prevent misdiagnoses is to consider the patient's life history in their cultural context.

Medicine's understanding is inherently tied to the individual patient, their specific circumstances, and the temporal and local factors involved. This perspective suggests that medicine may, in this aspect, be more aligned with the humanities than traditional science. However, it is worth noting that the distinction between science and humanities is not as clear-cut in all cultural traditions, and even within modern biology, the historicity and contextuality of phenomena are acknowledged [9, 10].

References

1. Mayr E. This is biology—the science of the living world. Cambridge: Harvard University Press; 1998.
2. Lawrence C, Weisz G, editors. Greater than the parts. Holism in biomedicine 1920–1950. New York: Oxford University Press; 1998.
3. Good BJ. Medicine, rationality, and experience: an anthropological perspective. Cambridge: Cambridge University Press; 1996.
4. Cassell E. The place of humanities in medicine. New York: Hastings Center of Society Ethics and the Life Sciences; 1984.
5. Engel GL. From biomedical to biopsychosocial. Being scientific in the human domain. Psychosomatics. 1997;38:521–8.
6. Pellegrino E, Thomasma D. A philosophical basis of medical practice. New York: Oxford University Press; 1981.
7. Engeström Y. Developmental studies on work as a testbench of activity theory. In: Chaiklin S, Lave J, editors. Understanding practice: perspectives on activity and context. Cambridge: Cambridge University Press; 1993. p. 64–103.
8. Leiman M, Stiles W. Integration of theory: methodological issues. In: Säfvestad-Nolan I, Nolan P, editors. Object relations and integrative psychotherapy. Tradition and innovation in theory and practice. London: Whurr Publishers; 2002. p. 68–79.

9. Viljanen A-M. A culture of psychiatry and culture in psychiatry: pathologising ypsy culture. Suomen Antropol. 1999;4:114–30.
10. Toulmin S. Knowledge and art in practice of medicine: clinical judgment and historical reconstruction. In: Delkeskam-Hayes C, Gardell Cutter M, editors. Science, technology, and the art of medicine. Kluwer Academic Publishers; 1993. p. 231–49.

Chapter 21
Professional Responsibility

Medical ethics ensures that the practice of medicine is not only about diagnosing and treating diseases but also about providing care that respects the individual, upholds moral standards, and promotes the overall well-being of patients. It is a multifaceted framework that requires doctors to act with integrity, competence, compassion, and an unwavering commitment to the best interests of their patients.

Medical ethics encompasses a set of principles and guidelines that guide the behaviour and decision-making of healthcare professionals, particularly doctors. It serves as a moral compass in the medical field, ensuring that physicians provide the highest quality care while upholding fundamental values.

1. Trust: Trust is the foundation of the doctor–patient relationship. Patients must trust their physicians to act in their best interests and to maintain confidentiality.
2. Fiduciary Responsibility: Doctors have a fiduciary duty to their patients, meaning they must put their patients' interests above all else. This includes avoiding conflicts of interest and making decisions solely in the patient's best interests.
3. Professional Competence: Medical ethics demands that doctors maintain a high level of professional competence. They must continually update their knowledge and skills.
4. Caring: Physicians are expected to show empathy and compassion towards their patients.
5. Mindfulness: Mindfulness in medicine refers to the ability of doctors to be fully present and attentive to their patients. It involves active listening, thorough examination, and a holistic understanding of the patient's needs and concerns.
6. Virtues: Virtues such as integrity, honesty, and empathy are integral to medical ethics. Doctors are expected to embody these qualities in their interactions with patients and colleagues.
7. Attitudes: A positive and respectful attitude is crucial in medical ethics. Doctors should treat all patients with respect and dignity, regardless of their background, beliefs, or condition.

S. Abbas, *Medical Ethics*, https://doi.org/10.1007/978-981-96-9199-9_21

8. Professionalism: Professionalism in medicine includes punctuality, confidentiality, ethical guidelines, and respectful interactions with colleagues and other healthcare providers.

   Core issues in responsibility, which are more than desired values.
9. Respect the sanctity of human life and the inherent dignity of each person.
10. Reject any involvement in or endorsement of crimes against humanity, firmly condemning such actions.
11. Provide competent and compassionate care to the sick and injured without bias.
12. Offer our expertise and skills when necessary, even if it entails personal risk.
13. Safeguard the privacy and confidentiality of those under our care, breaching this trust only in cases of severe danger to their well-being or that of others.
14. Collaborate openly with colleagues to explore, develop, and champion medical and public health advancements that alleviate suffering and enhance human welfare.
15. Educate the public and policymakers about existing and potential threats to human health.
16. Advocate for societal, economic, educational, and political reforms that alleviate suffering and enhance human welfare.
17. Guide and mentor the next generation of healthcare professionals, recognising that they represent the future of our caring profession .
18. Ensure patient safety and minimise harm [1].

> Professional competence is the habitual and judicious use of communication, knowledge, technical skills, clinical reasoning, emotions, values, and reflection in daily practice for the benefit of the individual and community being served. —Epstein and Hundert [2]

The definition serves as an entry point for understanding what professionalism is. It signifies that professionalism is not a single, straightforward concept but rather a multifaceted and complex set of behaviours, values, and principles.

The phrase "Professionalism in medicine" underscores the unique and heightened expectations placed on medical professionals. In the field of medicine, professionalism is not just a matter of competence but also encompasses a deep commitment to the well-being and welfare of patients. It involves a moral obligation to maintain the highest ethical standards, empathy, and integrity.

In the realm of medicine, professionalism takes on added significance due to the life-and-death nature of healthcare. Patients place immense trust in their healthcare providers, and professionalism is the cornerstone of this trust. It encompasses:

Ethical Decision-Making: Upholding moral values and ethical guidelines when making complex decisions about patient care.

Competence: A commitment to continuous learning and staying up-to-date with the latest medical knowledge and technologies.

Compassion: Demonstrating empathy and a caring attitude towards patients, even in challenging circumstances.

Communication: Maintaining clear and honest communication with patients, their families, and fellow healthcare professionals.

Confidentiality: Respecting and safeguarding patient confidentiality and privacy.

Collaboration: Collaborating effectively with colleagues and other healthcare providers for the benefit of the patient.

Patient Advocacy: Advocating for the best interests of the patient, including making difficult choices when necessary [2].

Professionals have a common dedication that unites them. Self-regulation is a hallmark of a profession, and physicians achieve this through state medical boards, hospital committees, and peer-review organisations. A profession has a reciprocal agreement with society.

During a patient encounter, we consider the most appropriate course of action, based on scientific and clinical evidence, for that individual. A compassionate approach factors into the patient's values and preferences.

Diagnostic Inquiry: This step involves understanding the patient's condition, history, exam, labs, and other data.

Therapeutic Assessment: We consider treatment options based on scientific evidence, including potential interventions.

Prudent Decision-Making: In this phase, it is important to share decision-making with the patient.

The Medical Professionalism Project, launched by the American Board of Internal Medicine Foundation, the American College of Physicians Foundation, and the European Federation of Internal Medicine, resulted in a 2002 professionalism charter. This charter outlined three core principles:

Patient Welfare: Emphasizing altruism, trust, and patient interest, and stating that external factors should not compromise this principle.

Patient Autonomy: Encouraging honesty, patient education, and empowerment for making informed medical decisions.

Social Justice: Highlighting physicians' societal commitment and consideration of available resources and the needs of all patients while caring for individual patients [3].

Teaching professionalism concepts can be challenging. Simply listing professional traits can be overwhelming. Additionally, students must grapple with negative media depictions of physician characters exhibiting unprofessional behaviour, such as on Grey's Anatomy, House, M.D., and Scrubs. To address this some American institutions begun incorporating segments from these shows into our discussions.

A significant issue in medical education is the "hidden curriculum." Despite an institution's defined values, individuals within it may sometimes display unprofessional behaviour, contradicting educational goals. Students start medical school with idealism, aspiring to become compassionate, capable doctors. However, this idealism often wanes. Research using moral reasoning assessment has revealed that medical students, upon completing medical school, tend to exhibit more cynicism than their nursing counterparts. The hidden curriculum impacts students distancing themselves from patients beyond professional boundaries, diminishing reflective thinking in favour of rote actions guided by specialty expectations, accepting hierarchical structures, and adopting specialty-specific physician identities.

Another challenge is that rating medical students on professionalism using a scale from 1 to 9 without additional feedback is not very constructive. A more effective approach is to employ a behaviour-focused method when instructing professionalism. Measuring values is complex and using value-related language in feedback can be intimidating. Values are often seen as innate and unchangeable. In contrast, behaviours are observable and quantifiable, which makes it less intimidating to point out deviations and provide specific corrective actions for students to improve their conduct. The focus moves from values to behaviours, but the fundamental values remain. Effective feedback not only clarifies the "what" but also delves into the "why," circling back to the underlying values. However, by first addressing behaviours, educators can access more information and have a stronger foundation to take action.

Medical students need to learn both cognitive and non-cognitive skills. Educators can assess cognitive skills like data collection, procedural competence, management, and use of technology. In contrast, professionalism relies on non-cognitive abilities, which include communication (language, empathy, integrity, compassion), collaboration (responsibility, respect, duty), and ongoing self-improvement (acknowledging limitations and striving for betterment) [4].

Teaching Professionalism

Numerous studies have indicated that teaching professionalism encompasses several stages:

Establishing clear expectations.
Conducting assessments.
Addressing inappropriate conduct.
Proactively averting such behaviour.
Fostering a shift in organisational culture.
Unacceptable behaviours can be written into policy statements.
Role modelling should be incorporated at all levels.
The consequences of inappropriate behaviour should be explained.
Equally crucial is outlining procedures, including reporting avenues, protecting whistleblowers from reprisals, remediation steps, and subsequent follow-up.
Final comprehensive evaluations, involving input from peers, nurses, patients, and diverse colleagues, hold particular significance, especially in assessing professionalism. While attending physicians may confidently assess a learner's knowledge and clinical decision-making, they might not be privy to their conduct during late-night situations.

Provision of remediation comprises the prompt recognition of undesirable behaviours. It entails holding a meeting to clarify acceptable standards and construct a well-defined remediation strategy. The potential repercussions for not demonstrating improvement should be clearly stated, including probation and dismissal.

Continuous follow-up is essential in all instances to monitor progress, acknowledge improvements, and explore avenues for ongoing enhancement [4]. Medical students who displayed unprofessional conduct during their time in medical school faced a threefold higher likelihood of facing disciplinary actions. This was particularly evident in cases of "severe irresponsibility" as per the code of conduct [5].

References

1. https://www.ama-assn.org/delivering-care/public-health/ama-declaration-professional-responsibility.
2. Epstein RM, Hundert EM. Defining and assessing professional competence. JAMA. 2002;287(2):226–35.
3. American Board of Internal Medicine Foundation. American College of Physicians–American Society of Internal Medicine Foundation. European Federation of Internal Medicine Medical professionalism in the new millennium: a physician charter. Ann Intern Med 2002;136(3):243–6.
4. Kirk LM. Professionalism in medicine: definitions and considerations for teaching. Proc (Bayl Univ Med Cent). 2007;20(1):13–6. https://doi.org/10.1080/08998280.2007.11928225. PMID: 17256035; PMCID: PMC1769526.
5. Papadakis MA, Teherani A, Banach MA, Knettler TR, Rattner SL, Stern DT, Veloski JJ, Hodgson CS. Disciplinary action by medical boards and prior behavior in medical school. N Engl J Med. 2005;353(25):2673–82.

Chapter 22
Patient-Centred Care

Patient engagement is a multifaceted concept that revolves around encouraging and enabling patients to play a proactive role in their healthcare journey. It extends far beyond the passive recipient of care to encompass a spectrum of actions and attitudes that empower individuals to assume responsibility for their health and healthcare. This active involvement may include a variety of activities, such as participating in shared decision-making, adhering to treatment plans, adopting healthy lifestyle choices, and gaining knowledge about their conditions.

Incorporating patients into decision-making processes is fundamentally rooted in the Nuremberg Code, which initially established and delineated informed consent as a prerequisite for involving individuals in therapeutic or research endeavours. Informed consent revolves around the principle that individuals must be fully informed and comprehend the nature of their involvement, as well as the associated risks and benefits.

At its core, patient engagement is about fostering a collaborative relationship between patients and healthcare providers. This collaboration involves open communication, trust, and mutual respect, with both parties actively contributing to the decision-making process. It acknowledges that patients possess valuable insights into their own experiences and preferences, which can significantly inform the course of their care.

The importance of patient engagement lies in its potential to enhance the quality of healthcare and improve patient outcomes. When individuals are engaged in their care, they are more likely to follow prescribed treatments, make informed choices, and actively manage their health conditions. This can result in better health outcomes, increased patient satisfaction, and ultimately, more efficient healthcare delivery.

Overall, patient engagement is increasingly recognised as a fundamental component of modern healthcare, underlining the shift from a paternalistic model of care to a more collaborative, patient-centred approach. It signifies a departure from the traditional, passive role of patients and represents a fundamental transformation in how healthcare is both delivered and experience.

S. Abbas, *Medical Ethics*, https://doi.org/10.1007/978-981-96-9199-9_22

Our primary attention will be directed towards addressing the patient engagement and health literacy requirements in three distinct scenarios: (1) decision-making, (2) health behaviour modification, and (3) the management of chronic diseases [1].

Patient Engagement

1. Take control of one's health and address health issues independently.
2. Participate in activities that mitigate the worsening of their condition or health deterioration.
3. Play an active role in making decisions about treatment and diagnosis.
4. Work closely with healthcare providers and caregivers.
5. Choose healthcare providers and organisations based on their performance, quality, or specific requirements.
6. Effectively navigate the healthcare system.

Importance

A number of recent studies have documented that organised care trials involving active patient engagement for chronic disease management led to substantial reductions in mortality when compared to control groups that solely adhered to appropriate medications. Patient engagement is the main component of value-based healthcare, to improve the quality of care while reducing its cost.

Engaging and activated patients who collaborate with their clinicians contribute to the promotion of health and well-being through improved care management. Furthermore, patient engagement marks a shift from paternalistic care models to collaborative partnerships between clinicians and patients. This partnership aims to enhance medical decision-making, educate patients about health and condition management, create systems for patient activation, and maintain patient involvement in their care. This implies that patients should have autonomy and play a central role in (a) ethics, as it upholds patient autonomy and self-determination, (b) interpersonal relationships, as it fosters confidence and trust in the clinician-patient dynamic, and (c) education, as it enhances knowledge, sets realistic expectations, and reduces decision-related conflict [2, 3].

It is important to realise the vital role of clinician communication styles in achieving effective patient engagement. "Good" communication fosters an atmosphere of unhurried interactions, a sense of clinician-patient understanding, and a trustworthy partnership. Learning effective communication is essential for all clinicians to engage a diverse range of patients with varying health literacy levels.

Clinicians are encouraged to begin with the presumption that all patients might face challenges in comprehending their health conditions and how to manage them.

Subsequently, clinicians should confirm and facilitate patients' understanding. Achieving full patient engagement across the healthcare continuum hinges on the patient's capacity to access, digest, and convey health information [4].

Patients who actively engage in their decisions tend to experience greater satisfaction with their care, acquire enhanced knowledge about their conditions, tests, and treatments, develop more realistic expectations about potential outcomes, exhibit higher adherence to screening, diagnostic, or treatment plans, experience reduced decision-related conflict and anxiety, receive fewer unnecessary tests or procedures, and, in certain instances, achieve improved health outcomes [5].

Key Factors

There are seven essential components for informed decision-making: (1) delineation of the patient's role in decision-making, (2) examination of the clinical matter at hand, (3) exploration of available alternatives, (4) evaluation of the advantages and disadvantages of these alternatives, (5) addressing uncertainties, (6) gauging the patient's comprehension, and (7) delving into patient preferences [6].

Challenges

1. Communication and language: Enhancing Communication Strategies. Utilising virtual visits and secure text messaging platforms Leveraging tele-health technology with multilingual support. Providing language translation services. Engaging caregivers in the communication process. Delivering training for improved interpersonal communication (eliminating medical jargon, adopting a slower pace, ensuring comprehension, asking relevant questions, etc.). Emphasising the significance of nonverbal communication and body language-Health literacy.
2. Enhancing Health Literacy Approaches: Tailored condition-specific educational videos Interactive quizzes to reinforce learning, offering patient-preferred educational formats (demonstrations, visuals, brochures, videos, one-on-one instruction, checklists, etc.), sharing appointment notes for clarity, assessing patient knowledge and addressing misconceptions Involving family members and caregivers and facilitating patient comprehension of symptom trends.
3. Addressing Social Determinants of Health (SDOH): Utilise SDOH screenings for assessment, recommend cost-effective dietary choices, establish partnerships to connect patients with affordable food and housing solutions, arrange medical transportation services, explore tele-health as an alternative to in-person care and mitigate social isolation issues.
4. Building Patient Trust Strategies: prioritise empathy and non-verbal communication, facilitate patient engagement through access to the patient portal, deliver

culturally sensitive care, foster a non-judgmental atmosphere, refraining from "medical fat shaming" or any form of patient demeaning, maintain transparency in discussing treatment and prognosis, educate staff to recognise and address bias [7].

Motivational Interviewing leverages patients' values and aspirations to initiate and sustain behaviour change. It's a "patient-focused approach that enhances inner motivation to change by addressing mixed feelings." Patients can develop this inner drive by connecting behaviour change with their identity, family and community roles, and personal values. Tailored patient education and support can increase self-confidence, explaining disease progression and the impact of behaviour changes on health. Relating behaviour change to personal experiences can reduce shame and guilt, offering hope for achievable change [8].

To enhance engagement design, clarify objectives, roles, and expectations for patients and caregivers. Specific roles and formal structures like steering committees or enabling patients to set agendas and participate throughout the process improved outcomes and maintained engagement. These techniques were used in mental health, HIV, and paediatric service settings to improve care access and quality. Training sessions were valuable in paediatric, diabetes, and home care contexts increasing confidence, and building positive relationships among users and staff. Training also helped mediate provider skepticism about patient engagement and power-sharing, promoting a more balanced partnership [9, 10].

Authors also supported flexible approaches to engage patients. Some employed various methods such as peer reporter interviews, headline generation, structured group discussions, written exercises, and questionnaires to gather patients' preferences. Other studies suggested involving a higher proportion of patients to amplify their voice. Regular updates to patient support groups were used to broaden patient involvement and address concerns informally. In one innovative approach, a buddy system was implemented to ensure user and family participation in mental health service quality improvement projects [11, 12].

Studies in general medicine, diabetes, mental health, and emergency services stressed the need for a receptive context achieved through balanced stakeholder representation. This was facilitated through techniques such as deliberation, democratic dialog, values and beliefs exercises, and narratives to foster shared understandings and an egalitarian spirit.

Ensuring equal user participation throughout the intervention-building process helped address power imbalances inherent in professionally delivered services. Location played a role in participation, with some consultations held outside the hospital setting or in community venues.

External facilitation was crucial in creating a receptive context that encouraged user involvement. It helped establish a positive working environment characterised by mutual respect and equal partnership. Additionally, attention was given to the physical environment, cleanliness, chair arrangement, and the use of props and visual aids to enhance discussions, interactions, and underscore the value of service users' contributions [13, 14].

Leadership played a pivotal role in successful engagement through various approaches, such as top-down strategies and local champions leading initiatives. This commitment was evident in mental health, HIV, and paediatric care settings and ensured organisational sustainability of engagement efforts. Ongoing contact with management and executives, along with an open attitude toward changes, demonstrated an ideological and policy commitment to meaningful involvement in. The timing of engagement, occurring before decision-making rather than providing input on already committed proposals, was stressed in multiple studies [4, 15]. patient experiences in the engagement process are diverse, with both positive and negative aspects. These experiences are influenced by factors such as the perceived impact of their involvement, the level of decision-making authority granted to them, and the amount of support and recognition they receive from the healthcare organisation [9].

Key Issues in Patient Engagement

Patient-Centred Care: where patients actively seek greater value from their interactions with providers. Patients are motivated to take a more active role in managing their health, and healthcare organisations are prioritising the patient experience to ensure consistent care throughout the journey.

Technology Integration plays a significant role in enhancing patient engagement. Patients now expect 24/7 access to digital platforms and intuitive online experiences, mirroring their on-demand access to various services like entertainment and social media access.

Emphasising Patient Education: Patients value health-related knowledge and actively seek an understanding of their health. Healthcare organisations are responding by delivering tailored and consistent education that goes beyond traditional handouts, recognising that patient engagement goes hand in hand with education.

Prioritising Patient Experience: As healthcare transitions to a more consumer-centric model, organisations are focusing on providing personalised, on-demand services that cater to the patient's needs.

References

1. Krist AH, Tong ST, Aycock RA, Longo DR. Engaging patients in decision-making and behavior change to promote prevention. Stud Health Technol Inform. 2017;240:284–302. PMID: 28972524; PMCID: PMC6996004.
2. Darkins A, Kendall S, Edmonson E, Young S, Stressel PM. Reduced cost and mortality using home telehealth to promote self-management of complex chronic conditions: a retrospective matched cohort study of 4,999 veteran patients. Telemed J e-Health. 2015;21(1):70–6.

3. Committee on Quality of Health Care in America and Institute of Medicine. Crossing the quality chasm: a new health system for the 21st century, Washington, DC: National Academy Press; 2001.
4. Elwyn G, Laitner S, Coulter A, Walker E, Watson P, Thomson R. Implementing shared decision making in the NHS. BMJ. 2010;341:c5146.
5. Stacey D, Legare F, Col NF, Bennett CL, Barry MJ, Eden KB, et al. Decision aids for people facing health treatment or screening decisions. Cochrane Database Syst Rev. 2014;2014(1)
6. Braddock CH 3rd, Edwards KA, Hasenberg NM, Laidley TL, Levinson W. Informed decision making in outpatient practice: time to get back to basics. JAMA. 1999;282(24):2313–20. https://doi.org/10.1001/jama.282.24.2313.
7. www.healthrecoverysolutions.com/resources/eguide/patient-engagement-guide#:~:text=Patient%20engagement%20describes%20the%20process,and%20partnering%20with%20healthcare%20providers.
8. Miller RW, Rollnick S. Motivational interviewing: preparing people to change addictive behavior. New York: The Guilford Press; 1991.
9. Weinstein J. Involving mental health service users in quality assurance. Health Expect. 2006;9(2):98–109.
10. Swarbrick MP, Brice GH Jr. Sharing the message of hope, wellness, and recovery with consumers psychiatric hospitals. Am J Psychiatr Rehabil. 2006;9:101–9.
11. Gibson F, Aslett H, Levitt G, Richardson A. Follow up after childhood cancer: a typology of young people's health care need. Clin Eff Nurs. 2005;9:133–46.
12. Murphy L, Wells JS, Lachman P, Bergin MA. Quality improvement initiative in community mental health in the Republic of Ireland. Health Sci J. 2015;9(13):1–11.
13. van Staa A, Jedeloo S, Latour JM, Trappenburg MJ. Exciting but exhausting: experiences with participatory research with chronically ill adolescents. Health Expect. 2010;13(1):95–107.
14. Iedema R, Merrick E, Piper D, Britton K, Gray J, Verma R, Manning N. Codesigning as a discursive practice in emergency health services: the architecture of deliberation. J Appl Behav Sci. 2010;46(1):73–91.
15. Cawston PG, Mercer SW, Barbour RS. Involving deprived communities in improving the quality of primary care services: does participatory action research work? BMC Health Serv Res. 2007;7:88.

Chapter 23
Duties of the Physician

The World Medical Association (WMA) is dedicated to upholding high ethical standards in global medical practice since its founding in 1947, following a grave violation of medical ethics. It has created essential documents to guide the medical profession, including the Declaration of Geneva (DoG), Declaration of Helsinki (DoH), and International Code of Medical Ethics (ICoME) [1].

The DoG, reaffirmed in 2017, sets out fundamental ethical principles for physicians. The DoH, last revised in 2022, addresses ethical challenges in medical research involving human subjects and is applicable to non-physician researchers.

The ICoME, established in 1949, outlines ethical principles and professional duties for the medical profession. These core documents are regularly reviewed and updated to maintain their relevance.

In 2018, a WMA international workgroup with members from diverse regions embarked on reviewing the ICoME, last revised in 2006. They consulted local ethics committees and experts to address outdated or missing ethical principles. The workgroup ensured that the ICoME accommodates diverse cultural and political contexts by considering linguistic nuances and regional interpretations. The effort to make the ICoME culturally inclusive and comprehensive was a collective one. The International Code of Medical Ethics should be viewed as a cohesive document, with each paragraph taken into account alongside others. While this Code is primarily directed at physicians in line with the WMA's mission, it is encouraged that all healthcare professionals also embrace these ethical principles [1, 2].

Physicians confront unprecedented challenges due to evolving clinical, political, legal, and market factors. Simultaneously, the medical field is becoming more interconnected globally, underscoring the importance of reaffirming the fundamental and universally applicable principles of medical ethics as outlined in the ICoME. The WMA and its members aim to boost awareness of this document through their advocacy efforts. By doing so, they aspire to establish a shared ethical framework for the medical community and reinforce professional identity.

S. Abbas, *Medical Ethics*, https://doi.org/10.1007/978-981-96-9199-9_23

General Principles

1. Physicians are primarily dedicated to advancing individual patient health through competent, timely, and compassionate care while upholding medical standards and professionalism. They must also consider their role in promoting public health, including future generations, while respecting human life, dignity, and patient autonomy.
2. Medical practice should be impartial and nondiscriminatory, based solely on patients' health needs, and should not show bias against factors such as age, disease, creed, ethnicity, gender, nationality, political affiliation, race, culture, sexual orientation, social status, or any other criteria.
3. Physicians should use healthcare resources efficiently to maximise patient benefits while practicing responsible resource management.
4. Honesty, integrity, accountability, and independent professional judgment are fundamental in medical practice, with physicians maintaining the highest standards of professional conduct.
5. Physicians must avoid conflicts of interest and not allow personal gain to influence their medical judgment, declaring and managing such conflicts when unavoidable.
6. Medical decisions should be based on sound professional judgment and not be altered due to non-medical considerations.
7. Physicians should collaborate with other healthcare professionals, ensuring patient confidentiality and sharing necessary information in the patient's best interest.
8. Professional certifications should only validate what the physician has personally verified.
9. When possible, physicians should provide aid during medical emergencies, taking into account their own safety and competence, as well as available care alternatives.
10. Physicians should never engage in or support acts of torture or inhuman treatment.
11. Continuous learning is essential for maintaining and improving professional knowledge and skills throughout a physician's career.
12. Physicians should aim for environmentally sustainable medical practices, minimising health risks to both present and future generations [1–3].

Duties to the Patient

1. The physician respects the patient's dignity, autonomy, and rights, including the right to accept or refuse care based on personal values and preferences.
2. The physician prioritizes patient well-being, striving to minimize harm and achieve a balance between intended benefits and potential harm.

3. The physician ensures the patient is fully informed, obtaining voluntary informed consent before any care is provided, and respecting the patient's right to withhold or withdraw consent.
4. When patients have limited decision-making capacity, the physician involves them as much as possible, considering their preferences and working with trusted representatives when available. Decisions are made in the patient's best interests when preferences cannot be determined.
5. In emergencies without a readily available representative, the physician may initiate intervention in the patient's best interests and respecting known preferences, if any.
6. If the patient regains decision-making capacity, informed consent for further intervention is obtained.
7. The physician communicates with those close to the patient, considering patient preferences, best interests, and confidentiality.
8. When a physician lacks the necessary capacity for a specific aspect of care, consultation or referral to a qualified colleague is ensured.
9. Accurate and timely medical documentation is maintained.
10. The physician upholds patient privacy and confidentiality, even posthumously, disclosing confidential information only under specific ethical obligations and with minimal necessary disclosure.
11. Patient awareness is maintained when reporting to third parties, with disclosure of commitments and consent obtained.
12. The physician refrains from inappropriate advertising or marketing and ensures factual, non-misleading information.
13. Professional judgment remains unbiased by commercial or financial interests.
14. Remote medical care is provided with medical justification, patient consent, and confidentiality protection, with direct contact preferred when suitable.
15. Professional boundaries are maintained, prohibiting abusive, exploitative, or inappropriate relationships with patients.
16. Physicians are responsible for their health and well-being, seeking appropriate care to ensure safe practice.
17. This Code represents the physician's ethical duties. In cases of profound moral dilemmas, conscientious objection may be exercised without harm or discrimination to the patient's health.

The patient must be informed of the objection and their right to consult another physician promptly [2, 3].

Duties to Colleagues and Personnel

1. The physician collaborates respectfully and without bias with other physicians, health professionals, and personnel, ensuring adherence to ethical principles when working in teams.

2. The physician respects colleagues' patient–physician relationships, intervening only when requested or when necessary to protect the patient from harm. Recommending alternative courses of action in the patient's best interests remains encouraged.
3. The physician reports conditions or circumstances hindering the provision of high-standard care or adherence to this Code to the relevant authorities. This includes reporting abuse, violence against healthcare personnel, inappropriate working conditions, or excessive and sustained stress-inducing situations.
4. Teachers and students are afforded due respect by the physician [3].
5. The physician must adhere to, safeguard, and champion the ethical principles outlined in this Code. Additionally, the physician should work to prevent the enactment of national or international requirements that contradict any of the obligations outlined in this Code.
6. The physician should assist and stand by fellow physicians in fulfilling the responsibilities established in this Code, ensuring their protection against unwarranted pressure, mistreatment, exploitation, violence, or suppression.

Duties to Society

1. The physician must advocate for fair and equitable healthcare, addressing disparities in health, the factors contributing to these disparities, and the rights of patients and healthcare professionals.
2. Physicians have a significant role in health-related matters, health education, and health literacy. When discussing medical advancements, technologies, or treatments in non-professional, public forums like social media, physicians must provide accurate and comprehensible information. They should indicate any personal opinions conflicting with evidence-based scientific data.
3. The physician supports ethical medical research following the WMA Declaration of Helsinki and the WMA Declaration of Taipei.
4. The physician should not engage in actions that undermine public trust in the medical profession. Upholding the highest professional standards and reporting unprofessional conduct to the relevant authorities are essential to maintaining this trust.
5. The physician shares medical knowledge and expertise to benefit patients and advance healthcare, public health, and global health [4].

References

1. Parsa-Parsi RW, Ellis R, Wiesing U. Fifty years at the forefront of ethical guidance: the world medical association declaration of Helsinki. South Med J 2014;107(7):405–406. https://doi.org/10.14423/SMJ.0000000000000127.

2. World Medical Association Declaration of Geneva. May 2006. https://www.wma.net/policies-post/wma-declaration-of-geneva/. Accessed 1 Sept 2022.
3. Parsa-Parsi RW. The international code of medical ethics of the world medical association. JAMA. 2022;328(20):2018–21. https://doi.org/10.1001/jama.2022.19697.
4. World Medical Association. WMA International code of medical ethics. 2022. Available: https://www.wma.net/policies-post/wma-international-code-of-medical-ethics/.

Chapter 24
The Informed Consent in Surgery and Medicine

Preconditions: Competence Voluntariness Informational elements: Disclosure of infromation Recommendation of a care plan Understanding of this infromation by th patient Consent Elements: Decision by patient Authorization by the patient to proceed

The concept of informed consent has predominantly been presented using the terminology of both legal and moral philosophy.

Informed consent finds its origins in diverse fields, spanning health professions, legal, and moral philosophy domains. Due to the legal system's retrospective and adversarial characteristics, the concept of informed consent for treatment has adopted a defensive tone. In this ethical framework, the primary justification for informed consent is based on the patient's right and capacity to make decisions that align with their values and desires. From an ethical viewpoint, the physician's duty to provide information is seen as a foundational element that enables patient autonomy, rather than being the central emphasis of informed consent.

Informed consent in medicine is a fundamental ethical and legal requirement that ensures patients have the necessary information to make educated decisions about their treatment or surgical procedures. This process involves comprehensive communication between healthcare providers and patients to ensure transparency, respect for patient autonomy, and protection from unwanted interventions. Informed consent in the context of medicine and surgery relies on the following principles:

S. Abbas, *Medical Ethics*, https://doi.org/10.1007/978-981-96-9199-9_24

1. The Principle of Autonomy
   Informed consent is rooted in the principle of patient autonomy, which upholds an individual's right to make decisions about their own healthcare.
   Patients have the right to be fully informed about the potential risks, benefits, and alternatives to a proposed treatment or surgery.
2. Components of Informed Consent
   Explanation of the diagnosis, including the nature and purpose of the treatment or surgery.
   Discussion of potential risks and benefits associated with the proposed procedure.
   Presentation of alternative treatment options, including the option of no treatment.
   Opportunity for the patient to ask questions and seek clarifications.
   Assurance that the patient's decision will not affect the quality of care they receive.
3. Competence and Capacity
   Healthcare providers should assess the patient's competence to make medical decisions. Patients must have the mental and emotional capacity to understand the information provided.
   In cases where a patient lacks capacity (e.g., due to mental illness or cognitive impairment), a legal guardian or surrogate decision-maker may provide consent.
4. Shared Decision-Making:
   Informed consent is not just about obtaining a signature on a form; it's a shared decision-making process.
   Healthcare providers should engage in meaningful discussions with patients, addressing their concerns, values, and preferences.
5. Voluntariness:
   Patients should feel free from coercion or pressure when making their decisions. They should be given adequate time to deliberate and should not be rushed into consenting.
6. Documentation:
   The informed consent process is documented in writing. Patients typically sign a consent form to indicate their agreement.
   The consent form should include the specifics of the procedure, potential risks, alternatives, and the fact that the patient has been given an opportunity to ask questions.
7. Exceptions:
   In certain emergency situations where obtaining informed consent is not feasible, healthcare providers may proceed with treatment to save a patient's life or prevent serious harm. However, they must later inform the patient or their family.
8. Ongoing Process:
   Informed consent is not a one-time event. It is an ongoing process, especially for complex or lengthy procedures.
   Patients should be kept informed of any significant developments or changes in their treatment plan.

9. Ethical Considerations:
   Ethical considerations, such as respecting cultural differences and ensuring that information is presented in a way the patient can understand, are integral to the informed consent process.

Informed consent in medicine is a fundamental ethical and legal requirement that ensures patients have the necessary information to make educated decisions about their treatment or surgical procedures. This process involves comprehensive communication between healthcare providers and patients to ensure transparency, respect for patient autonomy, and protection from unwanted interventions. Informed consent in the context of medicine and surgery relies on the following principles:

1. The Principle of Autonomy:
   Informed consent is rooted in the principle of patient autonomy, which upholds an individual's right to make decisions about their own healthcare.
   Patients have the right to be fully informed about the potential risks, benefits, and alternatives to a proposed treatment or surgery.
2. Components of Informed Consent:
   Explanation of the diagnosis, including the nature and purpose of the treatment or surgery.
   Discussion of potential risks and benefits associated with the proposed procedure.
   Presentation of alternative treatment options, including the option of no treatment.
   Opportunity for the patient to ask questions and seek clarifications.
   Assurance that the patient's decision will not affect the quality of care they receive.
3. Competence and Capacity:
   Healthcare providers should assess the patient's competence to make medical decisions. Patients must have the mental and emotional capacity to understand the information provided.
   In cases where a patient lacks capacity (e.g., due to mental illness or cognitive impairment), a legal guardian or surrogate decision-maker may provide consent.
4. Shared Decision-Making:
   Informed consent is not just about obtaining a signature on a form; it's a shared decision-making process.
   Healthcare providers should engage in meaningful discussions with patients, addressing their concerns, values, and preferences.
5. Voluntariness:
   Patients should feel free from coercion or pressure when making their decisions. They should be given adequate time to deliberate and should not be rushed into consenting.
6. Documentation:
   The informed consent process is documented in writing. Patients typically sign a consent form to indicate their agreement.

The consent form should include the specifics of the procedure, potential risks, alternatives, and the fact that the patient has been given an opportunity to ask questions.

7. Exceptions:
   In certain emergency situations where obtaining informed consent is not feasible, healthcare providers may proceed with treatment to save a patient's life or prevent serious harm. However, they must later inform the patient or their family.
8. Ongoing Process:
   Informed consent is not a one-time event. It is an ongoing process, especially for complex or lengthy procedures.
   Patients should be kept informed of any significant developments or changes in their treatment plan.
9. Ethical Considerations:
   Ethical considerations, such as respecting cultural differences and ensuring that information is presented in a way the patient can understand, are integral to the informed consent process.
10. Legal Implications: Failure to obtain informed consent can have legal consequences, as it may be considered medical malpractice or a violation of a patient's rights.
    In summary, informed consent in medicine and surgery is a pivotal aspect of patient care, emphasising respect for patient autonomy and ethical practice. It is both a legal requirement and an ethical obligation that ensures patients are active participants in their healthcare decisions, leading to better patient–provider relationships and improved overall patient care [1].

Moral Concepts Patients tend to remember only about 50% of what they are told, with long consultations that will they will switch off and could miss important parts of the consultation.

Moral concepts play a significant role in the process of consenting to surgery. Here are some key moral concepts and principles that come into play when a patient is providing informed consent for surgery:

1. Autonomy:
2. Informed Decision-Making:
3. Beneficence:
4. Non-Maleficence:
5. Truthfulness and Honesty:
   Truth-telling and honesty are moral virtues that apply in healthcare. Patients have the right to receive truthful information about their condition and the surgical procedure.
   Healthcare professionals have a moral obligation to be honest and transparent when discussing the surgery's details.
6. Respect for Dignity:
   This includes respecting their values, beliefs, and personal choices.
   Consent discussions should consider the patient's cultural and moral values to ensure that their choices are respected.

7. Confidentiality:
   Maintaining patient confidentiality is a moral duty. Patients must trust that their personal and medical information will be kept confidential.
   When discussing surgical procedures and obtaining consent, healthcare providers should respect patient confidentiality.
8. Shared Decision-Making:
   Ethical healthcare practices promote shared decision-making between patients and healthcare professionals.
   The moral concept of shared decision-making ensures that the patient is actively involved in the decision-making process.
9. Cultural Sensitivity:
   Cultural competence is an ethical consideration, ensuring that patients from diverse cultural backgrounds receive respectful and culturally sensitive care. Understanding the patient's cultural and moral beliefs can help.

   For informed consent to be valid, certain conditions must be met:

1. The patient must have the legal capacity to provide consent.
2. The consent must be given freely, without any form of coercion or pressure.
3. Patient must be provided with comprehensive information regarding the condition and the available options. This includes a clear understanding of the advantages and disadvantages associated with each choice, and the opportunity to seek clarifications through questions. Healthcare providers are legally required to furnish patients with essential information to enable them to provide informed consent for treatment. This information must encompass all significant risks associated with the recommended treatment [2].

The law acknowledges situations in which an individual might be incapable of granting informed consent, such as when decision-making capacity is impaired, or where consent may not be necessary, as in emergency cases. However, except in the case of children, where the High Court has acknowledged the courts' authority to authorise treatment through *parens patriae* jurisdiction [3].

In medieval times, doctors would request a "hold harmless document" that aimed to absolve them of any future liability in the case of adverse outcomes following treatment. This legal concept can be traced back to Italian, French, and Middle Eastern archives as early as the fourteenth century. Interestingly, it is considered an early precursor to informed consent, although its primary purpose was to protect the doctor rather than the patient. The evolution of modern Informed Consent legislation took shape in subsequent centuries, transitioning from case-specific litigation to becoming a standard practice. Notably, there are some remarkable historical cases that are worth mentioning in this context. One such case occurred in the eighteenth century when a patient sued his doctor for re-fracturing his leg and for experimenting with a novel external fixating mechanism without the patient's informed consent. This 1767 trial, known as Slater vs. Baker and Stapleton, stands as the earliest documented example of an Informed Consent case [4].

The foundation of contemporary Surgical Informed Consent (SIC) began to take shape in the early twentieth century, particularly with advancements in anaesthesia and more invasive surgical procedures with considerable risk of complications and mortality. A significant milestone in this evolution occurred in the case of Mohr vs. Williams in 1905 when a woman granted consent for surgery on her right ear. However, during the operation, the surgeon discovered that her left ear also required repair. Subsequently, the surgeon faced a lawsuit and was found guilty due to the deviation from the preoperative agreement. The judge characterised this agreement as a contract that only auth [5].

Another pivotal moment in the development of SIC came in 1914, with the case of Schoendorff vs. Society of New York Hospital, presided over by Justice Benjamin Cardozo. In this case, a woman had consented to an abdominal examination under anaesthesia but had not agreed to undergo surgery. Nevertheless, the surgeon proceeded to remove a tumour, which led to a legal dispute initiated by the patient. Justice Cardozo's verdict laid a cornerstone in the establishment of the SIC concept, stating, "Every mentally sound adult has the right to decide what is done with their own body. A surgeon who performs an operation without the patient's consent commits an assault and is liable for damages." [6, 7]

After World War II, the atrocities conducted by Nazi concentration camp "doctors" without patient consent led to a strong public backlash. In response to the Nuremberg trials (USA vs. Karl Brandt et al.), the Nuremberg Code was established, marking a significant milestone in the evolution of the informed consent process for trials. This code outlines ten essential requirements for all human research studies [8].

In the 1957 UK case Bolam vs. Friern Hospital Management Committee, the focus was on which risks should be discussed with a surgical patient, resulting in a doctor-centred view. This established the reasonable standard that surgeons should inform patients of what other surgeons typically disclose, known as the Bolam principle. However, the 1972 Canterbury vs. Spence case marked a shift towards a patient-centred standard, mandating the explanation of all risks and alternatives for a procedure. This trial introduced the "reasonable patient standard" [9, 10].

In 1992, the Australian High Court overturned the Bolam principle in the Roger vs. Whittaker case, emphasising the importance of patient requests for specific information, even when risks were considered low by the doctor. The "reasonable doctor standard" has since become a secondary standard alongside the "reasonable patient standard" in most countries [11, 12].

Since the 1980 Truman vs. Thomas case, the informed consent process must also encompass the risks associated with "not acting or postponing." In this case, a woman who refused a Pap smear claimed ignorance of the risks, specifically the potential delay in detecting curable cancer [13, 14].

The concept of informed consent can be understood from two distinct perspectives. The first perspective revolves around the idea of autonomous authorisation for a medical intervention, in direct opposition to the traditional paternalistic approach where the physician acts solely in the patient's best interest.

The alternative conception of informed consent places greater emphasis on the legal and institutional aspects, requiring a valid consent before a medical procedure. In this view, informed consent is regarded as an institutionally or legally recognised authorisation, and its validity is contingent upon adherence to specific institutional rules and practices [15].

Ethical elements of informed consent:

Valid informed consent incorporates five elements:

1. *Voluntarism* (free from coercion and from unfair persuasions and inducements).
2. *Capacity:* In practice, it is presumed that adults possess decision-making capacity unless strong evidence suggests otherwise. Clinically, several criteria can be employed to evaluate a person's capacity, including their ability to make choices, understand relevant information, grasp the situation and its consequences, and rationally process the provided information. The strictness of this standard varies depending on the importance, complexity, and implications of the decision. Competence pertains to the patient's legal authority to make healthcare decisions. For instance, a 17-year-old might possess the capacity to make decisions for themselves but lack legal competence.
3. *Disclosure:* is about giving patients information to comprehend a procedure. This includes details about the treatment's nature, purpose, risks, benefits, and available alternatives. Information should be conveyed in a simple manner. Common complications, regardless of severity, must be explained, as well as less common but potentially serious risks.
4. *Understanding:* entails the patient comprehending and recognising the information's relevance to her specific situation. Law and ethics lack a clear consensus on what qualifies as adequate understanding. Generally, courts have not considered lack of understanding as grounds for invalidating informed consent. Instead, they typically rely on evidence of the information disclosed to assess whether the patient was sufficiently informed.
5. *Decision:* pertains to the patient granting permission for a physician to proceed with the recommended treatment. While consent forms help facilitate and record this authorisation, they should be viewed as a secondary component to the process involving discussions and negotiations between the patient and the physician about the proposed treatment [15–19].

Physicians should be urged to elucidate patients' objectives, offer suitable choices aligned with these objectives, and provide recommendations following the "deliberative model" of the doctor-patient relationship [18].

Limitations of Informed Consent

While informed consent is closely tied to the ethical principle of respecting individual's autonomy, it serves a valuable practical role in medical care. Informed consent can lead to improved patient-physician relationships, enhance a physician's understanding of the patient's condition, and promote better patient adherence to treatment recommendations.

Two notable limitations are associated with the informed consent model. The first limitation revolves around the limited choices available. For instance, patients with a range of treatment options may face insurmountable obstacles, such as a lack of medical insurance, rendering independent decision-making irrelevant. A similar challenge is encountered in specific medical institutions that contend with regulations that restrict their autonomy. These rules dictate elements of their daily routines, ultimately posing a challenge to autonomy. Such constraints cannot be effectively addressed through the application of informed consent [20].

The idea of informed consent originated in the United States, a nation with a rich history of valuing individuality and personal rights. While this framework aligns well with many Western societies, it may not universally apply to all cultures. In some regions around the world, prioritising community norms and family ties takes precedence over individual autonomy.

Cultural perspectives on truth-telling can differ. Some cultures emphasise positive thinking and communication, sometimes prioritising this over candid discussions, even if it means sacrificing complete truthfulness, particularly in patients with advanced cancer where the prognosis is poor.

Balancing these tensions can be achieved by reaffirming the fundamental goal of informed consent, which is to honour an individual's autonomy. Respecting autonomy might involve permitting individuals to entrust certain decisions to others if they so choose. In real-world situations, finding the right equilibrium between upholding autonomy and accommodating a patient's preferences for information and decision-making authority can be a challenging task [19].

Consent for Being Involved in Clinical Trials

In 1991, the Department of Health and Human Services in the United States introduced the Common Rule, a set of regulations for human subjects research that applies to most federally funded research projects. This document mandates the provision of eight essential pieces of information to the patient or their legally authorised representative. These elements include:

1. A statement explaining that the study is investigational, a description of the research and its objectives
2. A detailed overview of potential risks and benefits for participants and others
3. Information about viable alternatives
4. Clarification regarding the impact of research participation on confidentiality
5. A statement on injury compensation (for studies with more than minimal risk)
6. Details on how the subject can obtain answers to relevant research questions
7. An explanation of the voluntary nature of participation and the right to withdraw,
8. The Common Rule also outlines "optional" elements of informed consent, which should be disclosed when applicable, encompassing unforeseeable risks, withdrawal conditions, and consequences, potential additional costs, provision of study-related

information affecting continued participation, and an estimate of the number of subjects. For research involving greater than minimal risk, the Common Rule mandates written documentation of informed consent and designates institutional review boards (IRBs) as the primary overseers of research compliance [21].

Obtaining consent for research differs significantly from securing consent for standard clinical care. In a research study, the investigator has ethical obligations to the scientific objectives of the project. However, when research subjects are also patients in clinical trials, these obligations may conflict with the investigator's responsibilities as a clinician. Research participants may struggle to distinguish between the physician–patient and investigator–subject relationships. Many research subjects mistakenly believe that the primary goal of their clinical trial is individual benefit, despite the investigator's clear explanation that the trial's purpose is to generate new scientific knowledge and enhance treatments for future patients. Such misconceptions can obscure the inherent trade-offs between risks and knowledge in clinical research, posing a potential threat to the validity of informed consent [22].

The principles of voluntarism, capacity, disclosure, and understanding are fundamental to informed consent, whether in research or medical treatment. Special attention is given to these concepts, especially voluntarism, and capacity, to provide additional regulatory safeguards for "special populations." Vulnerability among subjects can arise from specific situations or cognitive impairments. While these categories may intersect, prisoners are considered vulnerable due to their circumstances, whereas children and individuals with mental disabilities are considered vulnerable due to cognitive impairments. Under this category are, children, prisoners, and cognitively disabled people, patients with life-threatening illness, patients disadvantaged by socioeconomic and educational circumstances [23]

Informed consent serves as a crucial legal and ethical safeguard for healthcare providers, including surgeons. It primarily protects the surgeon in the following ways:

1. Documentation of Patient's Decision: providing patients with detailed information about the proposed treatment or surgical procedure, including its risks, benefits, and alternatives.
2. Mitigating Legal Liability: Informed consent helps to mitigate surgeons legal liability by demonstrating they informed the patient adequately. This can be a valuable defence against medical negligence claims.
3. Patient's Autonomous Decision: Informed consent upholds the principle of patient autonomy, which means the patient has the right to choose their own healthcare.
4. Promoting Trust and Transparency: Open communication during the informed consent process builds trust between the patient and surgeon. When patients are well-informed, they are more likely to cooperate and make fewer claims.
5. Educational and Ethical Value: It reinforces the importance of providing patients with comprehensive information, which is a fundamental ethical obligation.
6. Protection Against Claims of Battery: Without informed consent, performing a surgical procedure on a patient is a battery, which is an intentional tort.

It is essential for surgeons to ensure that the informed consent process is thorough and well-documented. Surgeons should take the time to answer the patient's questions and address any concerns to ensure that the patient fully comprehends the procedure and its associated risks. Ultimately, by respecting the principles of informed consent, surgeons can enhance patient safety, maintain professional integrity, and protect themselves from legal and ethical challenges.

References

1. UN Convention on the Rights of Persons with Disabilities, opened for signature 30 March 2007, 999 UNTS 3 (entered into force 3 May 2008) ART 17.
2. Rogers v Whitaker (1992) 175 CLR 479.
3. Secretary, Department of Health and Community Services v JWB and SMB (Marion's case) (1992) 175 CLR 218.
4. Eng Rep. Slater vs. Baker and Stapleton, 1767 (Slater vs. Baker and Stapleton 95 Eng Rep. 860 (k.b. 1767)).
5. Supreme Court of Minnesota (1905) Mohr v. Williams (104 N.W. 12 Supreme Court of Minnesota).
6. Recent Decisions: Tort. assault and battery. Unauthorized surgical operation constitutes "assault and battery". Virginia Law Rev. 1927;13(6):505.
7. N.E. Schoendorff v. Society of New York Hospital, 1914 (106N.E. 93 (N.Y. 1914)).
8. Vollmann J, Winau R. Informed consent in human experimentation before the Nuremberg code. BMJ. 1996;313(7070):1445–9.
9. WLR Bolam vs. Friern Hospital Management Committee, 1957 (1 WLR 583).
10. Armstrong AP, Cole AA, Page RE. Informed consent: are we doing enough? Br J Plast Surg. 1997;50(8):637–40. https://doi.org/10.1016/S0007-1226(97)90510-5.
11. Katz J. Reflections on informed consent: 40 years after its birth. J Am Coll Surg. 1998;186(4):466–74. https://doi.org/10.1016/S1072-7515(98)00045-3.
12. Skene L, Smallwood R. Informed consent: lessons from Australia. BMJ. 2002;324(7328):39–41. https://doi.org/10.1136/bmj.324.7328.39.
13. P. Truman vs. Thomas, 1980 (611 P.2d 902 (Cal 1980)).
14. World Health Organization Staff. Promotion of the rights of patients in Europe. In: Proceedings of a WHO Consultation; 1995.
15. Beauchamp TL, Childress JF. Principles of biomedical ethics. 3rd ed. New York: Oxford University Press; 1989. p. 1–470.
16. Meisel A, Roth LH, Lidz CW. Toward a model of the legal doctrine of informed consent. Am J Psychiatry. 1997;134:285–9.
17. Wertheimer A. Coercion. Princeton, NJ: Princeton University Press; 1987. p. 1–336.
18. Drane JF. The many faces of competency. Hast Cent Rep. 1985;15:17.
19. Emanuel EJ, Joffe S. Ethics in oncology. In: Bast RC, Kufe DW, Pollock RE, et al., editors. Cancer medicine. 5th ed. Hamilton: B.C. Decker, Inc.; 2000. p. 1145–63.
20. Berg JW, Applebaum PS, Lidz CW, et al. Informed consent: legal theory and clinical practice. Oxford: Oxford University Press; 2001. p. 1–340.
21. U.S. Department of Health and Human Services. 45 CFR 46. Fed Regist 1991;56:28012.
22. Lederer SE. Subjected to science: human experimentation in America before world war II. Baltimore: Johns Hopkins University Press; 1995. p. 1–192.
23. Faden RR, Beauchamp TL. A history and theory of informed consent. New York: Oxford University Press; 1986. p. 1–392.

Chapter 25
Prevention of Ethical Violation

Medical codes of ethics and professionalism bind doctors to uphold essential medical values, encompassing patient care, altruism, truthfulness, competence, compassion, empathy, and respect for patient autonomy. These values underpin the essential doctor-patient relationships essential for the goals of medicine, which include healing, disease prevention, and alleviation of pain and suffering. Although it can be challenging to consistently adhere to these ethical principles in every patient interaction, instances of severe ethical transgressions seem to be relatively infrequent. Such breaches often remain hidden, but when they do surface, disciplinary actions offer reliable insights into their prevalence. To provide some context, in the United States approximately 5 in 1000 physicians face disciplinary measures from state medical boards each year, with only 1.1 in 1000 experiencing severe disciplinary actions such as license revocation, suspension, or surrender of their licence.

Egregious violations of medical ethics, such as those involving sexual abuse of patients, criminal or negligent prescribing of opioids, or performing unnecessary surgeries for profit, are some of the most serious transgressions within the medical profession.

Sexual Abuse of Patients: This involves any sexual misconduct by a healthcare provider toward a patient, and it is an extreme breach of trust and medical ethics. It includes any unwanted sexual advances, harassment, or assault occurring within the context of the doctor-patient relationship. Such actions not only inflict serious emotional and physical harm on patients but also undermine the integrity of the medical profession.

Criminal or Negligent Opioid Prescribing: Opioid prescription abuse, whether through criminal activities like illegal drug diversion or negligent prescribing practices, has contributed significantly to the opioid crisis. It endangers patients' lives, leads to addiction, and can have severe public health consequences.

Performing Unnecessary Surgeries for Profit: When physicians perform unnecessary surgeries primarily for financial gain, it violates the most fundamental principle of medical care—putting the patient's well-being first. Unnecessary surgeries can lead to physical harm, emotional distress, and increased healthcare costs. These

S. Abbas, *Medical Ethics*, https://doi.org/10.1007/978-981-96-9199-9_25

practices undermine the trust that patients have in their doctors and the healthcare system.

These egregious violations not only harm individual patients but also erode public trust in the medical profession as a whole. To maintain the integrity of healthcare and uphold ethical standards, it is essential for the medical community and regulatory bodies to take these issues seriously. This may include implementing rigorous oversight, disciplinary actions, and public awareness campaigns to prevent and address such violations. Ultimately, the medical profession must consistently reinforce the importance of ethical conduct, prioritise patient welfare, and adhere to the highest standards of professional integrity [2, 3].

Larry Nassar was a physician who specialised in sports medicine. His case serves as a stark reminder of the consequences when medical professionals abuse their positions of power and their patients.

LaRenowned gymnasts, particularly USA Gymnasia and Michigan State University, used their trust in Nassar as a respected sports physician to exploit young female athletes.

Egregious Violations: Nassar's egregious violations included sexually abusing hundreds of young female athletes under the guise of medical treatment. He engaged in invasive and unnecessary procedures, often without consent, all the while abusing his position of trust and authority. These actions constituted not only a breach of medical ethics but also criminal sexual abuse.

Impact: Larry Nassar's case brought to light the vulnerability of young female athletes in sports medicine. Many survivors courageously came forward to share their experiences, shedding light on the pervasive culture of silence and complicity around sexual abuse in sports.

Legal and Ethical Ramifications: Nassar was arrested, prosecuted, and sentenced to a lengthy prison term for sexual abuse and assault. His case also prompted significant legal and ethical repercussions for the institutions and individuals who enabled or failed to address his misconduct.

The Nassar case triggered a cultural shift, emphasising the need for greater accountability and transparency in healthcare. It highlighted the consequences of medical professionals abusing trust. Survivors' stories led to justice for their abusers and changes in how institutions handle abuse allegations [2, 4].

Numerous aspects of the Nassar case are typical in various severe ethical violations: the perpetrator was male, the violations were repetitive and driven by self-interest, there was a lack of effective oversight, and those who became aware of the misconduct failed to act decisively. Consequently, similar actions must be taken to detect such cases earlier and respond promptly, irrespective of the type of violation [5].

Proposed Plan

Members of the research team from Washington University School of Medicine (WUSM) conducted a systematic literature review on legal and disciplinary actions in the field of medicine. They collaborated with research librarians from the Washington University Schools of Law and Medicine [1].

1. Recruitment of Trainees, Physicians, and Staff Aligned with Positive Medical Values

Medical institutions, including medical schools and medical centres, should actively seek individuals at various levels, including medical students, residents, fellows, attending physicians, and staff, who exhibit a strong commitment to fundamental medical values. These core values encompass qualities such as patient care, altruism, competence, compassion, and respect for patient autonomy. The practice of proactively assessing prospective medical students, residents, fellows, and staff using personality tests aimed at identifying deficiencies is a subject of debate, with questionable effectiveness.

Instead, the emphasis should be on identifying individuals who wholeheartedly embrace these positive values, as this approach is more likely to further the goals of the medical profession. A substantial body of literature has elucidated the virtues and attributes associated with medical professionalism. While the assessment of professionalism may be an ongoing challenge, it is widely acknowledged that an effective evaluation should adopt a multifaceted approach. This approach could involve methods such as using standardised patients, and employing validated tests with realistic scenarios [6–8].

2. Fostering Leadership and Professional Integrity

Issues in medicine often stem from broader cultural aspects within healthcare institutions. Transforming national and institutional cultures to prioritise respect for all individuals can cultivate professionalism. Leaders play a central role in enforcing policies and addressing physician misconduct. Unfortunately, severe ethical violations are frequently overlooked.

To combat this, it is essential to empower medical students, residents, nurses, and others who witness and report unethical behaviour, ensuring their protection against potential retaliation. A culture of professional integrity can provide better safeguards for both patients and whistleblowers than existing laws. To achieve this, leaders must promptly and transparently investigate credible complaints while respecting privacy. They should not tolerate actions that jeopardise patient safety or create a hostile work environment.

Selecting medical leaders should consider their character, experience, and qualifications, with formal training to enhance their leadership skills. Leadership programs for physicians should include dedicated sessions led by experts in organisational psychology and human resources, focusing on the rationale and strategies for effectively addressing serious misconduct [9–11].

3. Enhance Physician Feedback

Research shows that physicians are more likely to modify their behaviour positively when presented with objective data comparing their performance to peers or receiving 360° feedback from various sources. There are three ways to provide this feedback effectively:

First, institutions can conduct comprehensive physician evaluations, gathering feedback from a wide range of sources including patients, caregivers, family members, supervisors, peers, allied health co-workers, and trainees. This feedback can drive positive behaviour change while maintaining evaluator anonymity.

Second, prescription drug monitoring programs (PDMPs) can do more than just track "drug-seeking patients"; they can also provide physicians with feedback on their prescription patterns compared to peers in their specialty. Third, encouraging medical consultants to offer feedback to referring physicians and vice versa can foster a sense of peer oversight, acting as a safeguard against severe ethical violations [12–14].

4. Strengthen Peer Oversight

Oversight goes beyond feedback; it involves a structured approach to observation, creating a sense of being monitored. Research suggests that peer oversight and group practices can help prevent severe practice violations. Here are three examples of enhanced oversight, building on existing systems.

First, medical societies can mandate peer reviews of cases involving invasive or high-risk procedures. We propose that all practitioners of such procedures participate in registries supported by medical societies.

Second, in settings like solo medical practices where in-person peer reviews are challenging, electronic medical records can facilitate remote peer review. Encouraging peer reviewers with Continuing Medical Education (CME) credits for their auditing contributions can be beneficial.

Third, for medically necessary intimate examinations, chaperones should be a default practice, with exceptions granted only upon the patient's request. In certain cases, it is recommended that physicians lose their right to practice independently following significant deviations from established care standards in the absence of peer oversight [15, 16].

5. Enhance Wrongdoing and Consequence Tracking

Accurate tracking of wrongdoing is crucial for patient safety and supports informed decisions by disciplinary committees, patients, and researchers. Tracking consequences allows for transparent evaluation by state medical boards and other disciplinary bodies.

To improve tracking quality:

Mandate state medical boards and reporting institutions to provide detailed case descriptions.

To establish connections between specific wrongdoing and corresponding disciplinary actions.

Create a national tracking system to monitor major disciplinary actions from medical school through graduate medical education to medical practice. This confidential database would serve investigative and adjudicative purposes and track minor violations and accusations.

Recognise negligent reporting, credentialing, privileging, and failure to report physicians under disciplinary review as potential legal causes of action when patients are harmed.

Provide legal protection to institutions sharing information in good faith regarding a physician's professional history.

Encourage the sharing of physician billing patterns between private insurers and the Centers for Medicare and Insurance companies to detect fraudulent behaviour [17].

6. Promote Consistency and Transparency Among State Medical Boards

There is currently a significant disparity in how state medical boards handle serious professional misconduct cases. In certain states, physicians often resume their practice even after facing severe disciplinary actions for egregious violations. Boards should make their disciplinary actions publicly accessible on their websites [18].

7. Prevent Individuals from Practicing Medicine in Cases of Egregious Violations

Individuals who display a lack of concern for others, show no remorse for causing harm, and engage in illegal activities do not align with the fundamental values of medicine and pose a severe risk to patients. Behaviours that contradict the goals of medicine should be addressed promptly and justly, similar to how gross incompetence is managed. To safeguard both patients and physicians, medical boards should possess and utilise the authority to permanently revoke or suspend medical licenses for initial egregious offences that contradict medicine's core values such as rape. They should also be able to take these actions for repeated minor offences after attempts at correction. Medical schools and institutions offering residencies and fellowships should likewise have the power to dismiss medical students, residents, and fellows in such cases [2].

8. Collaborate with Law Enforcement

Administrative review by state medical boards can be a less burdensome approach for investigating and resolving cases like sexual abuse when compared to criminal investigations. Boards have the authority to remove a physician from practice more quickly than criminal proceedings. Boards should investigate whether victims, such as those of sexual abuse, wish to cooperate with law enforcement to pursue criminal charges. Patient preferences to not press charges should be respected. It is imperative to provide well-trained liaisons to assist boards in investigating various criminal activities, such as unnecessary invasive procedures and sexual abuse, similar to the support they offer for probing inappropriate opioid prescriptions [2].

9. Educate Patients to Make Informed Choices

The responsibility for ensuring competent and professional medical service should not rest solely on patients. Patients should be empowered by being provided with written information about topics like the use of chaperones during intimate examinations and the proper conduct of well-woman exams. Patients should be informed about their right to seek a second opinion, especially if they have concerns about a procedure's medical necessity. Vulnerable patients should have access to patient advocates and consent monitors when considering invasive or high-risk procedures [2].

10. Advance Research into the Causes of Serious Ethical Violations

Understanding the root causes of egregious ethical violations in medicine is essential for effective prevention and remediation efforts. We propose collaboration between state medical boards and researchers to identify relevant data points for investigating and reporting cases.

Research should also investigate the gender disparities among those who commit egregious ethical violations and assess the impact of increased gender diversity in medicine, particularly in leadership positions within healthcare institutions [2, 15, 19].

References

1. American Board of Internal Medicine, American College of Physicians, Medicine EFoI. Medical professionalism in the new millennium: A physician charter. 2004.
2. DuBois JM, Anderson EE, et al. Preventing egregious ethical violations in medical practice: evidence-informed recommendations from a multidisciplinary working group. J Med Regul. 2018;104(4):23–31.
3. Heumann M, Pinaire B, Burger S. Bad medicine: on disciplining physician felons. Cardozo J o Confl Resolut. 2009;11:133–80.
4. Murphy D Four new complaints filed against Larry Nassar, including one dating to '92. ESPN 2017.
5. Judd A State secrets: system shields doctors' abuse nationwide, leaves patients in dark. The Atlanta Journal Constitution September 26, 2016.
6. Papadakis MA, Teherani A, Banach MA, et al. Disciplinary action by medical boards and prior behavior in medical school. N Engl J Med. 2005;353(25):2673–82.
7. Lifchez SD, Cooney CM, Redett RJ 3rd. The standardized professional encounter: a new model to assess professionalism and communication skills. J Grad Med Educ. 2015;7(2):230–3.
8. Goss BD, Ryan AT, Waring J, et al. Beyond selection: the use of situational judgement tests in the teaching and assessment of professionalism. Acad Med. 2017;92(6):780–4.
9. Schuchman M. Medical whistle-blower protection lacking. Can Med Assoc J. 2008;178:1529.
10. Teaching medical professionalism: Supporting the development of a professional identity. 2nd Cambridge: Cambridge University Press; 2016.
11. Hodges BD, Ginsburg SR, Cruess R, et al. Assessment of professionalism: recommendations from the Ottawa 2010 conference. Med Teach. 2011;33(5):354–63.
12. Donnon T, Al Ansari A, Al Alawi S, Violato C. The reliability, validity, and feasibility of multisource feedback physician assessment: a systematic review. Acad Med. 2014;89(3):511–6.

13. DuBois JM, Chibnall JT, Anderson EE, Eggers M, Baldwin KA, Vasher M. A mixed-method analysis of reports on 100 cases of improper prescribing of controlled substances. J Drug Issues. 2016;46(4):457–72.
14. Pichert JW, Moore IN, Karrass J, et al. An intervention model that promotes accountability: peer messengers and patient/family complaints. Jt Comm J Qual Patient Saf. 2013;39(10):435–46.
15. Arora KS, Douglas S, Goold SD. What brings physicians to disciplinary review? A further subcategorization. AJOB Empir Bioethics. 2014;5(4):53–60.
16. Studdert DM, Bismark MM, Mello MM, Singh H, Spittal MJ. Prevalence and characteristics of physicians prone to malpractice claims. N Engl J Med. 2016;374(4):354–62.
17. Morreim EH. Malpractice, mediation, and moral hazard: the virtues of dodging the data bank. Ohio State J Disput Resolut. 2012;27(1)
18. Wolfe SM, Williams C, Zaslow A. Public citizen's Health Research Group ranking of the rate of state medical boards' serious disciplinary actions, 2009–2011. Public Citizen; May 17 2012.
19. Rochon PA, Davidoff F, Levinson W. Women in academic medicine leadership: has anything changed in 25 years? Acad Med. 2016;91(8):1053–6.

Chapte 26
Special Issues

The use of a morphine pump for an ill patient is not inherently a form of euthanasia. A morphine pump is typically used to manage severe pain and provide comfort to patients, especially those who are in palliative care or facing terminal illnesses. The primary goal of this pain management is to alleviate suffering and improve the patient's quality of life.

Euthanasia, on the other hand, involves intentionally ending a person's life to relieve suffering, typically at the patient's request. It is a morally and legally complex issue with various forms and definitions, and its permissibility varies by jurisdiction and cultural beliefs.

The crucial distinction here is that the intent behind using a morphine pump is to manage pain and improve the patient's comfort, not to end their life. In cases where high doses of opioids like morphine are administered to manage pain, ethical guidelines and laws often require careful monitoring and attention to ensure that the intention remains focused on pain relief rather than causing death.

However, the ethical considerations around end-of-life care, including pain management, can be complex and sensitive. It is essential for medical professionals to adhere to established ethical and legal guidelines in their jurisdiction and to communicate openly with patients and their families about the goals and expectations of care.

While the use of a morphine pump for an ill patient aims to alleviate pain and suffering, it is not considered a form of euthanasia as long as the primary intention is pain management rather than intentionally ending the patient's life. The ethical boundaries may vary by jurisdiction and should be followed in each case.

S. Abbas, *Medical Ethics*, https://doi.org/10.1007/978-981-96-9199-9_26

Criminalisation of Medical Errors

The healthcare industry has been abuzz with a recent case in which a Tennessee nurse faced criminal charges, including reckless homicide, after mistakenly administering a paralytic instead of a sedative, ultimately leading to charges of criminally negligent homicide and gross neglect. Some argue that criminal prosecution for causing patient harm is justified, but the reality is that prosecuting well-intentioned healthcare professionals for inadvertent errors may not effectively protect the public.

While infrequent, cases of healthcare providers facing felony charges after patient deaths are not isolated events in the United States. Similar situations have arisen in different states and healthcare professions. These cases extend beyond the United States, with healthcare professionals facing charges of gross negligence manslaughter in various countries. The outcomes of these domestic and international felony cases have varied, including imprisonment, probation, overturned convictions, plea bargains, dropped charges, and not-guilty verdicts.

However, the inconsistent and non-standardised application of criminal law to fatal medical errors is evident. The ambiguous line delineating criminal conduct leaves healthcare providers uncertain about the consequences of their actions, which may not effectively deter "criminal" behaviour [1, 2].

Moreover, criminal cases have primarily focused on errors resulting in patient death, overlooking non-fatal or non-harmful healthcare errors. This bias toward the severity or outcome of errors fails to safeguard society against similar future errors. It penalises those unfortunate enough to experience fatal outcomes while disregarding human and system errors when the consequences are not fatal.

Throughout these cases, it is evident that healthcare providers, despite their best intentions, are fallible humans operating in complex systems within the high-risk realm of patient care.

Patient Harm and Flawed Healthcare Systems

The World Health Organisation highlights a stark reality: the risk of suffering harm during healthcare is estimated at 1 in 300, whereas the risk of harm during air travel is just 1 in one million. This unsettling fact emphasises that patient harm ranks as the 14th leading global cause of morbidity and mortality. In high-income countries like the United States, approximately 1 in 10 patients experience harm during their hospital care, with nearly 50% of these adverse events being preventable.

The root of many medical errors can be traced back to systemic deficiencies rather than the actions of individuals. These system-related issues encompass various aspects such as technology, environment, culture, and workflow intricacies. In response to these challenges, healthcare professionals often resort to implementing workarounds or safety bypasses to fulfil their responsibilities. These workarounds, including actions like overriding a medication dispensing cabinet, directly result from flawed systems, not deliberate recklessness on the part of clinicians.

Healthcare providers operating within these complex systems often have little, if any, control over the multitude of variables. Thus, assigning blame to an individual for an outcome primarily driven by systemic flaws is unlikely to yield substantial improvements in patient safety. Incarcerating a lone clinician does little to safeguard future patients from harm since it fails to address the latent system failures that underlie such incidents.

In the intricate landscape of healthcare, patient harm is more likely to occur when latent and active errors coincide. Latent errors involve concealed systemic design or procedural shortcomings that create conditions allowing an active error to manifest. For instance, consider the case of the Ohio pharmacist who dispensed a compounded medication incorrectly. His account of the event highlights various latent system failures, such as:

Routine computer maintenance delaying medication label printing, leading to a backlog of orders and staff feeling rushed.

Interdepartmental miscommunication exacerbating time pressures on staff.

Reduced staffing levels.
Absence of rest breaks.

A small, cluttered workspace with materials for compounding multiple medications for different patients, resulting in incorrect material assumptions [3].

This is not to diminish clinicians' accountability or responsibility—they bear a significant share. However, singling out and criminally charging the clinician in close proximity to a patient harm incident, the one who made the final and obvious error amidst a chain of latent system and active errors, does not effectively prevent the recurrence of similar active errors. In fact, the Institute for Safe Medication Practices (ISMP) documented cases eerily resembling the Tennessee incident, suggesting that such errors had been reported both before and after that event.

Focusing on low-hanging fruit and isolating an individual healthcare provider's actions from the intricate system context does not address the broader systemic issues that continue to endanger patients. For example, in the Colorado case mentioned earlier, the ISMP identified over 50 distinct system failures that allowed the error to unfold, go unnoticed, and ultimately reach a healthy newborn child, leading to his tragic death. Had even one of these failures not occurred, the accident might have been prevented, or the error could have been detected and corrected before reaching the infant. Thus, criminally prosecuting the healthcare provider closest to the patient's harm is an inadequate solution, considering the intricacies of the healthcare system, the numerous departments involved, and the interactions among clinicians working together to provide care to a single patient. Such an approach falls short of safeguarding society as a whole, which is the primary purpose of criminal law [4].

System Improvement

To safeguard patients, all aspects of healthcare—workarounds, errors, questionable decisions, and risky behaviours—must be systematically identified and scrutinised, irrespective of the outcome. This rigorous analysis aims to uncover opportunities to enhance the system and reduce, if not eliminate, the need for workarounds. The key to achieving this lies in rectifying systemic deficiencies by introducing redundancies (multiple layers of safety barriers) and "people-proofing" processes. These measures are designed to preclude the inevitable human errors from reaching and harming patients [5].

For a healthcare institution to shift from a reactive stance, where responses occur after patient harm is already inflicted, to a proactive approach, which identifies and addresses system issues and workarounds following near-miss incidents, frontline clinicians are instrumental. These clinicians, who deliver direct patient care and continually interact with the healthcare system, must feel at ease reporting near misses, close calls, errors, adverse events, and concerns to the organisation, such as the quality management department and leadership. However, despite encouragement from organisational leaders and quality management staff, such reporting is not always forthcoming due to fears, including the dread of self-incrimination, punitive repercussions from leadership, and more. A culture of blame and shame, lack of trust, time constraints, and heavy workloads can also impede open reporting. Creating a culture of psychological safety, devoid of punitive tendencies, and fostering trust that the institution will act on the shared information are essential within the healthcare system. Externally, it necessitates freedom from the fear of criminal repercussions.

According to several healthcare entities and professionals, the long-term consequences of criminally prosecuting healthcare professionals (HCPs) tend to result in more, not fewer, errors and patient harm. Criminal charges induce fear in clinicians, not only of potential criminal and civil legal action but also of the information disclosed in event reports and quality improvement activities being admissible in legal proceedings, potentially used against them to assign blame and identify fault. This fear discourages incident reporting, which is pivotal for identifying and rectifying systemic issues, ultimately leading to more patient harm [6, 7].

Criminal prosecution of clinicians can also deter current and prospective healthcare providers from their profession, as they fear losing their livelihood. The result is a shortage of bedside clinicians, creating unsafe conditions and reducing access to healthcare, which can further contribute to patient harm. This approach also inadvertently fosters the misguided notion that perfection in healthcare is attainable when, in reality, it is not. This expectation of perfection can lead to clinicians concealing errors due to shame, preventing organisations from being transparent with patients and families about adverse events, eroding trust, and leading to more civil litigation. Increased civil litigation arises from the perception of attainable perfection, which, in turn, promotes defensive medicine, involving additional and often unnecessary testing that can potentially harm patients [8].

Proponents of criminally charging healthcare providers for fatal errors sometimes equate it to charging distracted drivers who, with full knowledge, engage in reckless, unsafe, and illegal behaviour, and in doing so, disregard known risks. However, this analogy overlooks several important distinctions. Healthcare providers generally do not make conscious decisions to be reckless or to ignore significant and unjustifiable risks. Instead, they engage in normalised workarounds engrained in the organisation's system, often used by numerous clinicians. These clinicians may fail to see the potential risk due to the frequent occurrence of the workaround without error or underestimate it, deeming it a justifiable means to provide timely patient care. These workarounds, sometimes termed "at-risk" behavioural choices, result from complex, substandard systems. Automatically removing an individual clinician responsible for an inadvertent mistake does not address the underlying flawed system that necessitated the workaround. Consequently, the flawed system persists, permitting other clinicians to engage in the same workarounds. As such, the path to patient safety should focus on proactively improving system design, thus minimising the need for workarounds.

Accountability for Clinicians and Organisations

In a healthcare system that fosters a blame-free culture and psychological safety for incident reporting, accountability extends to both clinicians and organisations. These shared responsibilities include:

For Individual Clinicians

Maintaining mindfulness, presence, and focus during tasks.

Minimising distractions and errors during higher-risk work.

Avoiding assumptions and seeking clarification when necessary.

Recognising and rectifying at-risk behaviours.

Advocating to leadership about system issues that demand improvement.

Consistently reporting errors and near misses.

Actively participating in incident investigations and analysis.

Engaging in education, coaching, retraining, and remediation.

Encouraging open dialogue about incidents and their lessons.

For Healthcare Organisations.

Prioritising patient safety.

Cultivating a blame-free environment that encourages incident reporting.

Listening to clinician concerns and reported incidents.

Investing time and resources in investigating events and implementing improvements.

Proactively monitoring and acting on information from national patient safety organisations.

Analysing this information in the context of the organisation's processes and systems.

Devoting resources to reconcile any discrepancies and implement recommendations and best practices [9].

Exploring Alternatives to Criminal Prosecution of Clinicians

In light of the widespread system issues associated with fatal medical errors, various alternative approaches have been proposed to address the complexities inherent in such cases:

Corporate Manslaughter Charges: Some advocate for holding healthcare institutions and their leadership accountable through corporate manslaughter charges. This approach targets those responsible for directing and allocating resources within healthcare organisations in a manner that may lead to patient harm.

No-Fault System, Modelled After New Zealand: The implementation of a no-fault system, similar to the one in New Zealand, has gained support. This model recognises that the criminal law is often ill-suited to address the intricate interplay of error, violations, and systemic failures typically seen in cases resulting in prosecutions of healthcare professionals for gross negligence manslaughter.

Professional Licensing Boards: In light of the complexities involved in healthcare provision and the healthcare system, some suggest that a state's professional licensing board, composed of peers of the subject clinician, is a more appropriate and reliable avenue for evaluating care, investigating harm allegations, upholding professional standards, and determining suitable sanctions. This administrative route still prioritises public protection but is better aligned with addressing failures in clinical practice without implying criminal intent [10, 11].

In Conclusion

Recognising that errors are inherent when humans are involved, it is essential to acknowledge that the real root causes of harm in healthcare are flawed healthcare systems and latent failures that enable predictable human errors to reach patients. Criminalising these human errors does not rectify or prevent these underlying causes, nor does it adequately protect society and the patients relying on healthcare systems. In fact, it may lead to counterproductive long-term effects. Emphasising the imperfection of human practitioners operating within imperfect healthcare systems underscores the importance of focusing on the most reliable approach to prevent patient harm: continuous refinement and enhancement of the dynamic healthcare system.

References

1. Dyer C. Court overturns optometrist's conviction for gross negligence manslaughter. Br Med J. 2017;358:j3749.
2. Dyer C. Senior surgeon's conviction for manslaughter is quashed. Br Med J. 2016;355:i6178.
3. Patient Safety Network, Latent error (or latent condition) (n.d.). https://psnet.ahrq.gov/taxonomy/term/3488.
4. Institute for Safe Medication Practices, Lesson from Denver: Look beyond blaming individuals for errors (Feb. 11, 1998), https://www ismp.org/resources/lesson-denver-look-beyond-blaming-individuals-errors.
5. Philipsen NC. The criminalization of mistakes in nursing. J Nurse Pract. 2011;7(9):719–26. https://doi.org/10.1016/j.nurpra.2011.07.004.
6. Institute for Safe Medication Practices, Criminalization of human error and a guilty verdict: A travesty of justice that threatens patient safety (2022), https://www.ismp.org/resources/criminalization-human-error-and-guilty-verdict-travesty-justice-threatens-patient-safety.
7. Ameratunga R, Klonin H, Vaughan J, Merry A, Cusack J. Criminalisation of unintentional error in healthcare in the UK: a perspective from New Zealand. Br Med J. 2019;364:l706.
8. Marx, D., Reckless homicide at Vanderbilt?: A just culture analysis (2019), https://www.outcome-eng.com/wp-content/uploads/2019/03/Vanderbilt-Homicide-A-Just-Culture-Analysis_David-Marx.pdf.
9. Institute for Safe Medication Practices, 2016–2017 Targeted medication safety best practices for hospitals (2016), https://www.neomedinc.com/wp-content/uploads/2016/02/ISMP-2016-2017-TMSBP-for-Hospitals.pd_.pdf.
10. McCartney M. Clinical errors need a systemic response. Br Med J. 2018;360:k812. https://doi.org/10.1136/bmj.k812.
11. The American Association of Nurse Attorneys, TAANA position paper on Samuel's law executive summary (2015), https://taana.org/resources/Positions/samuel2015.pdf.

Chapter 27
Dehumanisation in Medicine

A Patient Not a Person

The foundational ethical principles of the medical profession encompass prioritising a patient's best interests, recognising patients as individuals with intrinsic worth, promoting patient autonomy in making informed treatment choices, and ensuring equitable access to medical benefits. The neoliberal market ideology, which views individuals as commodities and commercialises healthcare, has a detrimental impact that estranges healthcare providers from their patients.

A patient tells her physician, "I'm not merely a diabetic; I'm a person who also happens to have diabetes." Meanwhile, a nurse, engrossed in typing on a computer, mechanically inquires, "On a scale from one to five, please rate your pain." In another scenario, an African American man arrives at the emergency room displaying signs of a heart attack but is statistically less likely than a white patient with identical symptoms to receive a medication that can dissolve blood clots.

Dehumanisation of patients in medical care refers to the process by which healthcare providers or the healthcare system, intentionally or unintentionally, treat patients in a way that disregards their humanity, dignity, and individuality. It involves reducing patients to mere objects, medical conditions, or sets of symptoms, rather than recognising them as unique human beings with feelings, rights, and personal values.

Dehumanisation can happen in various ways, such as:

1. *Disregarding patient preferences*: Failing to involve patients in decisions or ignoring their values and preferences.
2. *Impersonal interactions*: Treating patients as case numbers rather than addressing them by name and establishing empathetic connection.
3. *Stereotyping*: Making assumptions about patients based on their age, gender, ethnicity.
4. *Lack of informed consent*: Administering medical treatments or procedures without obtaining the patient's clear and informed consent.

S. Abbas, *Medical Ethics*, https://doi.org/10.1007/978-981-96-9199-9_27

5. Poor communication: Using medical jargon or failing to communicate clearly, leading to misunderstandings.
6. *Neglecting emotional needs*: Focusing solely on the physical aspects of an illness while overlooking patients' emotional, psychological, and social well-being.
7. *Objectification:* Viewing patients as bodies with diseases rather than as people with physical, emotional, and social dimensions.

Dehumanisation in healthcare can have detrimental effects on patients, leading to dissatisfaction, mistrust, and even worse health outcomes. It is essential for healthcare providers and institutions to foster a patient-centred approach that respects the inherent dignity and humanity of every individual receiving medical care. Dehumanisation fundamentally involves the refusal to acknowledge the presence of a uniquely human mind in another individual. When considering the human mind, is generally described through two key facets: the ability to experience (including feeling pleasure and pain) and the capacity for agency (which encompasses planning, intention, and the exercise of choice) [2]. The denial of experience often leads to treating others as if they were unfeeling machines, while the denial of agency typically results in treating others as if they were uncivilised, irrational animals [3].

Dehumanisation is measured differently in various research studies. One approach examines infra-humanisation, a form of dehumanisation that involves withholding secondary emotions like nostalgia and humiliation from others. Importantly, these emotions rely on higher-order mental abilities, such as self-reflection and retrospection, or in terms of the denial of uniquely human traits (that involve logic, reason, and civility) or traits typical to human nature (that involve emotion and inter-personal warmth, While these diverse conceptualisations of dehumanisation may differ in their details, a common element among all of them is a reduced tendency to attribute and acknowledge the mental states of others, the process is unconscious, unintentional and non-malicious. Numerous scholars have contended that the field of medicine is progressively losing its human touch, as it becomes more dominated by impersonal technologies and economic considerations, which have put the physician patient relationship under unprecedented strain [3, 4].

The Dual Nature of Dehumanisation in Medicine

Dehumanisation in medicine serves both functional and nonfunctional roles. Some aspects of dehumanisation are essential for effective healthcare, while others are largely unnecessary and detrimental to patient care.

Functional Dehumanisation

Mechanisation, the process of viewing patients as physiological systems, is necessary for clinical problem-solving and targeting specific medical issues within the human body.

Empathy reduction, which allows medical professionals to maintain emotional detachment during high-stress situations, is crucial for effective problem-solving and efficient patient care.

Transient moral disengagement, which occurs when physicians must inflict temporary pain or discomfort on patients during medical procedures, helps medical professionals focus on the larger goal of treating pathology and returning patients to health.

Nonfunctional Dehumanisation

De-individuation practices, such as current dressing practices that lead to a loss of individuality, have little utility in medical contexts and may be detrimental to patient well-being.

Perceptions of impaired patient agency, which strip patients of their ability to make decisions and plan, do not benefit patient care and can be counterproductive.

Dissimilarities between patients and physicians, although they may exist due to differences in status and expertise, are not advantageous for patient involvement in their care.

It's important to note that even functional dehumanisation can have negative consequences when used outside of specific contexts where it is functional. Inappropriate mechanisation or empathy reduction can lead to patient alienation and mistrust. Moral disengagement can have harmful effects or encourage unnecessary procedures for personal gain. Therefore, functional dehumanisation in medicine should be approached with caution and used sparingly and judiciously in appropriate clinical settings [1, 2].

Underlying Causes

1. Mechanisation: Dehumanisation in medicine often arises due to the functional requirements of the profession. For example, medical diagnosis and treatment frequently necessitate a mechanistic approach, viewing patients as complex systems composed of interacting components, which leads to objectification, where individuals are seen as devoid of emotional responsiveness or interpersonal warmth. De-compartmentalising individuals into their constituent parts is helpful

for diagnosis and locating health issues. However, this practice inherently involves some level of dehumanisation in clinical contexts.

Furthermore, the process of breaking down individuals and their symptoms into physiological systems and subsystems is essential for effective problem-solving in medicine. This approach may often overlook patients' mental states, focusing on the physical aspects of the condition. Medical problem-solving tends to centre on specific aspects of the human body, potentially disregarding the patient's inner mental experiences [3].

2. Less empathy: non-physicians shed light on this phenomenon. Physicians exhibited significantly less brain activation in areas associated with empathy for pain but showed increased activation in regions related to executive control and self-regulation. Multiple factors contribute to physicians' reduced empathy, primarily stemming from their medical training. Medical training encourages the regulation of negative emotional responses to enhance efficient problem-solving, leading to dampened empathy. Research indicates that the neural networks involved in social cognition and nonsocial problem-solving are inversely correlated. Dehumanisation becomes more pronounced in demanding clinical situations where the pressure to provide efficient care is high. This may serve as a coping mechanism to manage stress. A paradoxical finding is that medical students initially report high levels of empathy in their first years but experience a decline as they have more direct patient interactions [5].
3. Moral Disengagement.

   Dehumanisation often arises from the need for medical professionals to momentarily detach themselves from the harm inflicted during procedures, even if it's necessary for treatment. This moral disengagement, which involves separating moral self-sanctions from inhumane conduct, serves to either justify past or prospective harm. Physicians find themselves in both contexts and may dehumanise patients to minimise guilt when causing pain, even if it's essential for treatment. Dehumanisation makes it psychologically easier to harm patients without personal distress.
4. De-individuating patients: Where individuals lose their distinctive identity in a group or through anonymisation. This can lead to dehumanisation in two ways: it can de-individuate the person being perceived (the dehumanised) or the perceiver (the dehumaniser). De-individuation may result in antisocial behaviour by diminishing feelings of personal responsibility for actions or by making the target less identifiable. Caregivers may dehumanise patients due to the de-individuation of the medical environment, where they become anonymous among colleagues. Patients, in turn, may also experience de-individuation, appearing as faceless entities among others seeking help, rather than individual agents in need of empathy. Racial or ethnic minority patients may face amplified de-individuation. When doctors view such patients as generic, hyper-de-individuated members of a minority group, it can result in unequal care [6].
5. Reduced Patient Agency: Is the perception of patients as having diminished agency. This form of dehumanisation emerges from the hospital setting, where many individuals have limited abilities to plan, intend, and take actions,

essentially diminishing their capacity as agents. The loss of agency often results from various medical conditions, including traumatic injuries, infections, drug use, chronic pain Even when patients genuinely have these limitations, focusing on these shortcomings can intensify a form of dehumanisation that resembles animalisation [2, 3].

6. Patient Dissimilarity: Arises from perceived dissimilarity between physicians and patients, which can manifest in three primary ways.

   First, illness inherently sets patients apart from the typical, well-functioning human, as it often alters appearance, behaviour.

   Second, the labelling of patients as their illnesses, like referring to someone as "a schizophrenic" rather than "a person with schizophrenia," exacerbates dehumanisation by implying that the person has become the disease itself, rather than a fundamentally human being affected by the disease.

   Third, the power imbalance in the doctor-patient relationship, where doctors often hold a superior position, can have a specific impact on dehumanisation, this is due to illness, which inherently involves a loss of power and control over their lives. Doctors' authority in this relationship can be a significant factor in dehumanisation, as it can create a sense of mastery over patient [2, 7].

Suggested Solutions

Individuation

To counter de-humanisation caused by de-individuation, steps can be taken to promote individuation and personalisation of doctors and patients. This can involve reversing practices that anonymise both parties and embracing strategies that foster identification and personal responsibility among physicians.

For instance, the tradition of healthcare professionals wearing uniform white coats can de-individuate physicians by making them seem less personally responsible for their actions. To enhance personal responsibility and individuation, caregivers and patients can abandon the practice of wearing group-specific uniforms like military cadets or soldiers. While these practices may be deeply rooted in tradition, considering the psychological aspects of dehumanisation reveals an irony: Certain traditions, like the "white coat ceremony," might unintentionally hinder medicine from combating de-individuation [2].

Promoting Similarity: There are various approaches to foster doctor-patient similarity, reducing dissimilarity as a source of dehumanisation. One fundamental way to achieve this is by increasing diversity among physicians in terms of race, ethnicity, and gender to better reflect the demographics of their patient population.

However, there was a significant discrepancy in terms of racial and ethnic representation.

It's important to note that physicians generally belong to one of the highest-earning professions and are substantially wealthier than the average citizen. Striving for demographic similarity alone can help reduce the perception of intergroup boundaries, which are often the basis for dehumanisation [4].

Medical education and training should include practices that encourage physicians to recognise the shared humanity they have with their patients. This can involve acknowledging their shared mortality, understanding illness narratives, and recognising vulnerability to disability, suffering, personal loss, and various forms of uncertainty. Furthermore, institutions should discourage the practice of labelling patients solely by their diseases and instead emphasise the patient's humanity. A combination of these efforts can effectively counteract dehumanisation stemming from the perception of patients as less human [7, 8].

Reorienting the Focus on Patient Agency: To address the issue of impaired patient agency, medical settings can take steps to refocus the attention of both doctors and patients on the patient's ability to plan and make choices.

One approach is to acknowledge and highlight the patient's past or present professional experiences, or entrusting patients with tasks like caring for a plant or involving them as active partners in clinical decision-making.

An experiment conducted in nursing homes demonstrated that providing patients with these simple reminders of their agency was associated with a significant increase in their lifespan [9].

To humanise the patient experience in healthcare, medical professionals can shift from using administrative identifiers like birthdates or Social Security numbers to more personal information.

During medical rounds and discussions, doctors can start by sharing details about the patient's personal history, such as their name, place of birth, profession, hobbies, and family life. Incorporating this personifying identification can serve as a reminder of the patient's humanity and help prevent dehumanisation.

In surgical procedures, a similar approach can be adopted. Before starting a surgery, medical teams can announce the patient's name and provide a brief narrative about their life, offering a humanising touch to the procedure.

Another strategy involves making patients' faces more visible during procedures, contrasting with practices like hooding or masking that induce dehumanisation in non-medical contexts. Transparent drapes could replace opaque ones, allowing patients to be seen and humanised. This approach may enhance patient care, reduce errors, and improve attention to detail [10].

Empathetic Balance and Physician Selection

Balancing empathy and cognitive objectivity is crucial for physicians. Empathy is valued by both doctors and patients, as it benefits patient outcomes. Physicians with higher empathy scores, as measured by the Jefferson Scale of Physician Empathy, produce better clinical results. Reduced physician empathy is linked to perceived medical errors, while patients who perceive their physicians as empathic are more likely to adhere to treatments.

To promote an effective balance between empathy and cognitive problem-solving, medical education should move away from prescribing a strict preference for either empathy or cognitive objectivity. Physicians need to recognise when to employ each approach, depending on the patient and the context. For example, surgeons may be more empathic in outpatient settings but require less empathy in the operating room.

To achieve this balance, medical schools need to consider interpersonal skills when selecting applicants. They can assess empathy using validated measures as these measures predict real-world empathic behaviour. Additionally, structured interviews like the Multiple Mini-Interview (MMI) can evaluate applicants' abilities in establishing trust, emotional responsiveness, effective collaboration, measured thinking, and handling disagreements.

Medical schools employing such methods have seen improved performance in doctors' decision-making, patient interactions, and cultural competency. This approach can help identify and cultivate physicians with the practical wisdom to optimise care through balanced empathy and cognitive problem-solving [10, 11].

Enhancing Moral Engagement and Reducing Dehumanisation

To combat the dehumanisation stemming from moral disengagement, it's essential to minimise the psychological distance between doctors and patients. One approach is to reevaluate patient dressing practices in hospitals, which currently can be humiliating and degrading. Patients often wear gowns that expose their private parts and may have designs that contribute to their humiliation. These clothing choices not only strip patients of their dignity but also create an unnecessary divide. Studies like the Stanford Prison Experiment have shown how degrading clothing can lead to brutal treatment of individuals.

Instead, medical settings should offer clothing that is practical for physical examinations without compromising the dignity of patients during their most vulnerable moments. This shift in attire can help bridge the psychological gap between medical professionals and patients, making patients appear closer and deserving of moral consideration.

The introduction of technology can also widen the psychological and moral gap, contributing to dehumanisation. Technology can create a sense of detachment, making it easier to perform actions with moral consequences. Physical contact between individuals is usually seen as a more morally significant act compared to actions mediated by technology.

Physicians often work with abstract representations of patient data and images. To counter this, including a patient's image with all medical records, can not only humanise the patient but also mitigate the potential for technology to amplify dehumanisation. This simple adjustment can serve as a reminder of the real human suffering behind the data and images and promote a stronger sense of moral engagement in medical practice [12, 13].

Dehumanization of patients during hospitalization highlights the need for proactive measures in hospital contexts. These measures should encompass the education of healthcare professionals, clinical practices, administrative policies, social interventions, and research.

At the clinical level, humanizing patients begins with taking their medical history, which fosters empathy and intercultural dialogue between healthcare and the humanities. Engaging with patients through their history facilitates a partnership in their care, enhances the therapeutic relationship, reduces stress, and strengthens their commitment to treatment. This approach also benefits the well-being and professional competence of healthcare providers.

Administratively, action against discrimination is essential. Strategies to address interdisciplinary discrimination can help alleviate health inequalities. These strategies should acknowledge the multifaceted nature of social identity and promote support and equality within healthcare services.

In medical education, incorporating humanities courses, communication skills workshops, and training in narrative techniques for medical history-taking can further promote patient-centred care and combat dehumanisation in healthcare settings [14–16].

References

1. Beauchamp T, Childress J. Principles of biomedical ethics. New York: Oxford University Press; 2001.
2. Dehumanization in Medicine: Causes, Solutions, and Functions Omar Sultan Haque and Adam Waytz. Harvard University and Northwestern University.
3. Haslam N. Dehumanization: an integrative review. Personal Soc Psychol Rev. 2006;10:252–64.
4. Leyens JP, Cortes BP, Demoulin S, Dovidio J, Fiske ST, Gaunt R, et al. Emotional prejudice, essentialism, and nationalism. Eur J Soc Psychol. 2003;33:703–17.
5. Hojat M, Mangione S, Cohen MJM, Gonnella JS, Erdmann JB, Veloski JJ, et al. The Jefferson scale of physician empathy: development and preliminary psychometric data. Educ Psychol Meas. 2001;61:349–65.
6. Jenni K, Loewenstein G. Explaining the "identifiable victim effect". J Risk Uncertain. 1997;14:235–57.
7. Kleinman A. The illness narratives: suffering, healing, and the human condition. New York: Basic Books; 1988.
8. Bursztajn HJ, Feinbloom RI, Hamm RM, Brodsky A. Medical choices, medical chances: how patients, families, and physicians can cope with uncertainty. New York: Routledge; 1990.
9. Langer E, Rodin J. The effects of choice and enhanced personal responsibility for the aged: a field experiment in an institutional setting. J Pers Soc Psychol. 1976;34:191–8.
10. Zimbardo PG. The Lucifer effect: understanding how good people turn evil. New York: Random House; 2007.
11. Harris G. New for aspiring doctors, the people skills test. New York Times. (2011, July 10).
12. Haslam N. Humanising medical practice: the role of empathy. Med J Aust. 2007;187:381–2.
13. Haney C, Banks WC, Zimbardo PG. Interpersonal dynamics in a simulated prison. Int J Criminol Penol. 1973;1:69–97.

14. Hauser MD, Cushman FA, Young L, Jin R, Mikhail J. A dissociation between moral judgments and justifications. Mind Lang. 2007;22:1–21.
15. Chadwick R. Compassion: hard to define, impossible to mandate. Br Med J. 2015;351:Article No. h3991. https://doi.org/10.1136/bmj.h3991.
16. Warner HJ. The humanizing power of medical history: responses to biomedicine in the 20th-century United States. Procedia Soc Behav Sci. 2013;77:322–9. https://doi.org/10.1016/j.sbspro.2013.03.090.

Chapter 28
How to Deal with Difficult Patients

The term "difficult patient" is a subjective and somewhat controversial term used in the medical and healthcare field to describe a patient who presents challenges or difficulties for healthcare providers. A "difficult patient" is not a specific medical diagnosis or condition but rather a description of a patient's behaviour, attitude, or circumstances that can make their care and treatment more challenging. Some common reasons a patient may be considered difficult include:

Non-Compliance: Patients who do not follow medical advice, treatment plans, or medication regimens can be seen as difficult because their non-compliance can hinder their recovery or management of their condition.

Demanding Behaviour: Some patients may exhibit demanding, entitled, or aggressive behaviour, making it challenging for healthcare providers to communicate effectively and provide care.

Complex Medical Conditions: Patients with complex medical issues, multiple chronic conditions, or rare diseases can be perceived as difficult due to the specialised knowledge and time required for their care.

Emotional or Psychological Issues: Patients with mental health conditions or emotional distress may exhibit behaviours that healthcare providers find challenging to address.

Unexplained Symptoms: Patients with persistent, unexplained symptoms that do not fit a clear medical diagnosis can pose challenges for healthcare providers in determining appropriate treatment.

Language or Cultural Barriers: Patients who have limited proficiency in the local language or come from different cultural backgrounds may face communication challenges with healthcare providers.

Substance Abuse: Patients with substance abuse issues may be challenging due to their health risks, non-compliance, or unpredictable behaviour.

It's important to note that labelling a patient as "difficult" can be stigmatising and may not be helpful in providing appropriate care. Healthcare providers are trained to address these challenges with empathy, understanding, and effective

S. Abbas, *Medical Ethics*, https://doi.org/10.1007/978-981-96-9199-9_28

communication. The term "difficult patient" is often discouraged in modern healthcare, and healthcare professionals are encouraged to focus on patient-centred care and finding ways to overcome barriers to effective treatment and communication.

Patient–provider interactions can be complex at times. We've all been part of consultations that did not go as smoothly as we would like, whether we were the healthcare provider or the patient. In such instances, neither party intends to create a challenging situation, but it often happens due to common misunderstandings on both sides. Effective communication and listening skills are crucial in all medical consultations, especially in cases where interactions might become challenging [1].

Examples of scenarios can include situations where a doctor:

1. Exhibits poor nonverbal communication during a consultation, such as avoiding eye contact with the patient, focusing solely on computer screens or notes, displaying negative body language, or using an inappropriate tone of voice.
2. Shares distressing news in an inappropriate setting, such as delivering bad news in a busy hospital corridor with onlookers like medical students and other patients.
3. Provides challenging information, such as a life-altering diagnosis, without displaying empathy or ensuring the availability of support services like counselling or the presence of caregivers/family members.
4. Communicates ambiguously, failing to explain long-term management plans or the significance of a diagnosis in plain language.

On the other hand, these scenarios can also occur when a patient:

1. Conducts online research about their medical condition and firmly believes in their findings, insisting on specific tests or treatments.
2. Feels unheard or frustrated during medical consultations, leading to potential threats of legal action or publicising their concerns on social media.
3. Refuses to adhere to recommended treatments, attending appointments with deteriorating health, such as a heavy smoker with severe asthma who continues to smoke and doubts the effectiveness of their inhalers.
4. Disagrees with the doctor's diagnosis or test results and requests a second opinion.
5. Experiences persistent symptoms impacting their quality of life, despite extensive evaluations by various medical teams, resulting in frustration or a loss of trust in healthcare providers.
6. Concentrates on past issues rather than focusing on the best way to move forward [1, 3].

To address and alleviate challenging interactions, it's crucial to consider the factors that contribute to such situations. Two key factors include the healthcare environment where these interactions occur and the differences in clinical practices across regions and countries. The majority of healthcare settings are grappling with excessive workloads and strained resources due to high demand, which significantly impacts these interactions.

Inadequate time for consultations or patient interactions is a critical element, given the mounting pressures on healthcare systems, and rising expectations, all set against a backdrop of cost-cutting. It is essential to keep in mind that both patients and healthcare professionals share the common goal of fostering a positive interaction, recognising the value of the time spent during consultations for all parties involved.

Every patient arrives at the clinic with a unique clinical and psychosocial history, which influences their behaviour. Their beliefs and expectations are shaped by their personality, the severity of their symptoms, and how these affect their quality of life.

Previous negative experiences and disappointments within the healthcare system can be challenging to overcome, fostering mistrust. These circumstances can create feelings of anxiety, worry, hopelessness, and uncertainty, sometimes manifesting as tension and negative reactions toward healthcare providers.

Patients may have high expectations and trust in the system, but when it seems that their condition has no clear solution or prognosis due to the disease's nature, it can be distressing. Language barriers, cultural diversity, can contribute to misunderstandings.

Furthermore, patients have various considerations to weigh, such as how their diagnosis might affect their other responsibilities (work, family, etc.). Many patients juggle work and other commitments, which the diagnosis may impact or has already influenced, delaying the timing of seeking help. It's crucial to remember that being defined solely by their diagnosis and labeled as "a patient" is not, and should not be, the sole aspect of their lives [2–4].

The Healthcare Provider

The development of effective communication skills among healthcare practitioners varies significantly, posing a notable challenge. Communication skills training is not consistently integrated into the specialist curriculum, and it is not a prerequisite for specialist post applications. Poor communication can result in Poor word choice and phrasing, often based on assumptions about the patient's understanding of medical concepts.

Lack of a structured approach when delivering challenging news, resulting in scattered information that confuses patients or no clear plan at all.

Selection of inappropriate settings for delivering difficult news.

Different options for treatment are not explained.

Limited involvement of the patient in the decision-making process, with treatment decisions made without considering their preferences.

Rushing the patient to agree to a proposed treatment plan.

Hasty interaction due to time constraints.

Neglecting to refer the patient to support services or resources like counselling, support groups, or reliable information sources online.

Breaking bad news may occur in an un-empathetic manner, healthcare professionals may discuss patient matters with nurses over the patient's head, using complex medical terms, which makes them feel excluded from the conversation. Routine clinical data for the provider can be overwhelming for the patient, creating an impression of coldness and a lack of empathy.

Time constraints in the clinic may lead to providers not listening to the patient's concerns, and overlooking vital questions about the patient's fears, information needs, and experiences. Additionally, the patient may not have the time to fully express their thoughts.

In complex clinical cases, doctors may become overly focused on solving the medical problem, neglecting the fact that the patient might be overwhelmed by anxiety, frustration, and negative emotions. Patients often require reassurance to feel safe, comfortable, and to trust their doctor.

The healthcare setting, whether an outpatient clinic or a hospital ward, is familiar territory for doctors to have difficult conversations. However, for patients, this setting can be uncomfortable and awkward, particularly when they are about to receive a diagnosis.

Furthermore, a doctor's emotions or behaviour may be influenced by factors such as sleep deprivation, personal health issues, job satisfaction, etc. The doctor's approach and communication style significantly impact their interactions and can have adverse effects on the patient, especially if the doctor comes across as arrogant or impatient and they don't take responsibility for discussing the situation with the patient in terms they can understand.

It's essential for doctors to recognise that some patients may feel intimidated by the imbalance in the doctor-patient relationship. This perception can be exacerbated when doctors behave in a condescending or patronising manner. Many of these challenges should be addressed through training and ongoing professional development [3–5].

Dysfunctional healthcare systems exacerbate the tensions between patients and doctors. Issues such as long waiting times at clinics, frequent appointment cancellations, as well as delays in prior appointments and medical investigations can all contribute to challenging interactions between patients and healthcare providers. Doctors often become the initial point of contact for patients when things go awry, exposing them to the immediate frustrations of patients.

Insufficient resources, including staffing levels and the maintenance of patient privacy and dignity during consultations, further contribute to this problem.

The absence of centralised documentation systems sometimes results in patients having to repeatedly provide the same information, diverting attention away from managing the clinical case and addressing the patient's needs. This constant repetition, especially when encountering new doctors, can lead to patient frustration and make it challenging for healthcare providers to gauge the patient's prior understanding [4–6].

The final outcome of a challenging situation has the potential to result in various consequences. For patients, this may manifest as growing concerns, frustration, feelings of vulnerability, uncertainty over the course of their treatment and prognosis, fear, worries, dissatisfaction, and a loss of confidence in the patient-doctor relationship, patients can feel they are not heard and consequently feel more vulnerable. They might have encountered negative experiences with hospitals or healthcare facilities in the past and maybe apprehensive that voicing concerns or inquiring about their treatment could lead to delays or other negative effects.

Conversely, for doctors, it can lead to heightened anxiety, anger, a sense of helplessness, and the adoption of avoidance strategies, such as discharging patients prematurely or sending them to another colleague.

These consequences also have broader implications for the healthcare system. They can lead to the misallocation of resources, and an increased demand for second opinions. This means that the patient will either try the "doctor shopping" approach or unnecessarily attend the emergency department.

Suggested Plan for Difficult Situation

Prepare for effective communication:

Plan ahead to deliver the news thoughtfully to the patient.
Choose words that are considerate and clear, breaking down complex i information.
Encourage patients to confirm understanding and summarise key points.

Foster open communication:

Avoid underplaying the challenges of the disease.
Involve the patient in treatment decisions and establish a cooperative approach.
Consider the role of the patient's partner or caregiver, especially during difficult discussions.

Ensure a conducive environment:

Select an appropriate setting and confirm audibility.
Obtain patient consent for observers.
Pay attention to nonverbal communication cues.
Provide support and resources:
Offer contact information for further questions.
Guide patients to reputable information sources.
Keep initial information simple and encourage note-taking.

Continuous improvement:

Discuss challenging cases with colleagues and seek additional training if needed.
Recognise individual differences in communication and adapt your approach.
Monitor signs of patient discomfort and adjust the conversation if necessary.

Build trust and rapport:

Prioritise patient psychological safety and open communication.
Address difficulties openly and find common ground.
Help patients regain emotional control and engage them in decision-making.
Highlight solutions and seek feedback:
Offer actionable options after summarising the situation.
Encourage questions and engage patients in decision-making.
Ask for patient feedback on the consultation experience.

Reflect and learn:

Analyse challenging interactions and identify areas for improvement.
See difficult situations as opportunities for learning.
Seek feedback from peers and supervisors [1, 7].

Set Clear Boundaries
While empathy and understanding are crucial, it's also essential to define and maintain clear boundaries when interacting with your patient. These boundaries outline the behaviours that are considered acceptable or unacceptable within your practice or at the hospital. Ensure your patient acknowledges and agrees to these boundaries.

Consider establishing a treatment plan with the patient where both parties agree on acceptable behaviours, such as you agree not to use offensive language when communicating with our care providers," or "I do not prescribe addictive medications." By involving the patient you can enhance their engagement with their care and strengthen your relationship.

Set Boundaries
It's essential to be aware of your own weaknesses when confronted with challenging interactions. Consider whether your skillset are well-suited to effectively handle the situation, or if it might be more appropriate to involve someone else to collaborate with. If the situation escalates to the point where the patient becomes physically or verbally abusive, it's time to take a step back. Clearly communicate to them that they have crossed a line, and their behaviour is unacceptable.

Recognise When to Conclude a Doctor-Patient Relationship
Assess the situation to determine if it is feasible to continue treating a patient when the trust within the relationship has eroded. It might be in the best interest of both the patient and yourself to discontinue their care.

Documentation
Exercise thorough care when documenting encounters, particularly those involving confrontations or difficult discussions with patients or their family members. Maintain an objective and factual summary of the interaction.

Self-Care and Support
Managing challenging interactions with patients and their families can be emotionally demanding. Prioritise not only the well-being of your patients but also that of your team. To effectively navigate these stressful encounters, it's essential to

maintain a healthy work-life balance. Additionally, seeking support and assistance from your colleagues can be highly beneficial.

Reflection

After a challenging interaction with a patient, take some time to reflect on the events and your responses. Consider the outcomes and the lessons learned from the experience, as this reflection can better prepare you for similar interactions in the future [1, 6, 7].

References

1. Hardavella G, Aamli-Gaagnat A, Frille A, Saad N, Niculescu A, Powell P. Top tips to deal with challenging situations: doctor-patient interactions. Breathe (Sheff). 2017;13(2):129–35. https://doi.org/10.1183/20734735.006616. PMID: 28620434; PMCID: PMC5467659.
2. Philip J, Kissane DW. Responding to difficult emotions. In: Kissane DW, Bultz B, Butow P, et al., editors. Handbook of communication in oncology an palliative care. New York: Oxford University Press; 2010. p. 135–46.
3. Jackson JL, Kroenke K. Difficult patient encounters in the ambulatory clinic: clinical predictors and outcomes. Arch Intern Med. 1999;159:1069–75.
4. Kreger J. When your patients are in mourning. FPM. 2003;10:49–50.
5. Epstein RM. Mindful practice. JAMA. 1999;282:833–9.
6. Edmondson AC. Learning from failure in health care: frequent opportunities, pervasive barriers. Qual Safety Health Care. 2004;13(Suppl. 2):ii3–9.
7. Bramson RM. Coping with difficult people. Garden City: Anchor Press/Doubleday; 1981.

Chapter 29
The Difficult Colleague

Today, the typical physician concludes their formal education armed with impressive technical skills for addressing bodily diseases. However, when it comes to tending to the human aspect of illness and patient care, their proficiency often relies on the innate abilities and personal qualities they possessed upon entering medical school. There exists a substantial body of knowledge on human behaviour accumulated since the turn of the century, with the potential to enhance patient care. Unfortunately, this wealth of knowledge remains largely unfamiliar to them. Neglecting this crucial dimension of a physician's education underlies patients' frequent complaints about physicians being insensitive, callous, neglectful, arrogant, and mechanical in their approach [1].

Throughout medical school and residency, students and residents frequently encounter challenges involving not only their supervisors but also peers and support staff. Difficulties can also emerge when collaborating with colleagues for patient care and consultations, potentially contributing to physician burnout. Moreover, we contend that every physician, over the course of their career, dedicates a significant portion of their time to navigating challenging relationships with colleagues, The terms "impaired," "disruptive," and "problematic," in addition to "difficult," were employed as adjectives to categorise doctors or physicians who are difficult to deal with [1].

The Impaired Doctor

The expression "impaired doctor" typically denotes the most severe cases of atypical behaviour, which may involve conditions like psychosis, cognitive dysfunction, or problems related to drug addiction. An impaired doctor typically pertains to a situation where a physician is deemed incapable of fulfilling their professional responsibilities, often because of factors like mental or physical health issues.

S. Abbas, *Medical Ethics*, https://doi.org/10.1007/978-981-96-9199-9_29

Certain countries have established obligatory guidelines for reporting impaired doctors [2, 3].

The Disruptive Doctor

The term "disruptive doctors" has various interpretations, with Reynolds emphasising that it shouldn't be applied to physicians expressing controversial ideas or constructive criticism of the medical system. The American Medical Association (AMA) and the organisation responsible for hospital accreditation define disruptive behaviour encompasses "personal conduct, whether verbal or physical, that negatively affects or has the potential to affect patient care, including any conduct that hinders collaboration with the healthcare team. However, well-intentioned criticism aimed at enhancing patient care is not considered disruptive behaviour." The organisation responsible for hospital accreditation characterises disruptive doctors as those engaged in "intimidating and disruptive behaviours, including overt actions like verbal outbursts and physical threats, as well as passive behaviours like refusing assigned tasks or silently displaying uncooperative attitudes during routine activities [4, 5].

The operating room and emergency department present a challenging work environment marked by its high complexity and workload. Surgeons leading procedures must collaborate effectively with the surgical team to ensure smooth interactions. The existing but limited research indicates that disruptive behaviours may be more prevalent among surgeons, as well as interventional physicians, and doctors practicing in emergency departments [6].

Examples of disruptive behaviours include using crude language and swearing, not being available when on call, consuming alcohol or drugs on duty, making discriminatory remarks towards minority colleagues, engaging in sexually harassing comments or actions with colleagues, staff, and trainees (such as unwanted advances and offensive language), spreading false information about a colleague's integrity, creating divisions within the treatment team, failing to meet responsibilities in a passive-aggressive manner, excessively using projection, and threatening litigation during performance reviews or when confronted with complaints about their behaviour, (90%) of the "disruptive doctors" were diagnosed with a personality disorder [7, 8].

The Problem Doctor

The term "problem doctor" is employed in two distinct ways. Some articles narrowly define "problem doctors" as those with subpar clinical skills, while other definitions are broader and encompass physicians involved in sexual offences, or disruptive behaviour. Research on the prevalence of physicians exhibiting problematic behaviours is limited. Notably, sexual misconduct is an area that has garnered significant attention within psychiatry. Female physicians were underrepresented among troubled physicians. Psychiatrists were nearly twice as likely as non-psychiatrists to face disciplinary action for engaging in sexual relationships with patients, and they were also charged with negligence and incompetence at a similar rate. The remedy for these problems is addressed in professionalism [8–10].

Challenging Physicians" from the Physician's Viewpoint

Doctors may be hesitant to discuss their colleagues from this perspective. Such reticence could be attributed to the medical profession's traditional code of ethics, which places a strong emphasis on respecting fellow physicians. Additionally, the prevailing approach to medical education, often characterised as "tacit learning" under the guidance of physician mentors, seldom encourages physicians to question the thought processes of their peers. While most doctors would concur that "impaired physicians" or "disruptive physicians" should face disciplinary actions when necessary to safeguard patients [11].

Communication Challenges among Physicians

Communication challenges among physicians can be attributed to two primary factors. The first factor encompasses persistent patterns of negative behaviour displayed by some physicians, which psychiatrists often classify as personality disorders. The second factor pertains to situational issues linked to trust, clinical decision-making, and collaborative interactions with consulting colleagues [1]. In psychiatry, the diagnosis of personality disorders is made when "personality traits manifest as enduring patterns of perceiving, relating to, and thinking about the environment and oneself, and are consistently displayed across a variety of significant social and personal situations [12]. In 1985, Gabbard, a psychoanalyst, suggested that physicians may commonly exhibit compulsiveness, which is characterised by doubt, guilty feelings, and an exaggerated sense of responsibility, the prevalence is not known with surgeons admitted to significantly elevated levels of narcissism. Narcissism and arrogance, which result in an inflated self-image of the physician, can lead to a belief that they know better than their colleagues or consultants. This can disrupt the workflow within healthcare organisations [13].

The original Hippocratic Oath emphasises the importance of intellectual humility and respect for colleagues and their opinions, which are fundamental in clinical practice. When individuals become overly focused on their perceived accomplishments, professional success, or institutional roles, it can foster arrogance and lead to a lack of respect for those in different positions [14, 15].

A constructive approach to addressing the topic of "disruptive doctors" is to centre the discussion around "empathy". Those with minimal or no "empathy" often struggle in medical fields that involve patient interactions but excel in procedure-oriented specialties. On the other hand, some individuals possess a higher level of "empathy" but may misuse it to "manipulate" others rather than genuinely aiding them [16].

Situational Problems

Situational factors that can disrupt physician communication encompass trust issues, disparities in clinical judgment, and interactions with consultants [1].

Trust

In the patient–doctor relationship, there are five dimensions: (a) expectations of competence, (b) the degree of concern doctors have for patient welfare, (c) physician authority in decision-making, (d) physician management of confidential information, and (e) physician willingness to provide and receive information. These same dimensions apply to relationships among physicians, spanning a spectrum from the assumption of colleague competence and adherence to established norms to complete distrust necessitating ongoing vigilance. Problematic doctors may be colleagues with whom trust has eroded due to repeated negative experiences, or physicians who have difficulty trusting anyone and insist on maintaining full control. Inadequate communication regarding patients and care responsibilities, gaps in clinical knowledge, superficial interactions, and misunderstandings can undermine trust [17].

Disparities in Clinical Judgment

The challenge of inconsistent clinical judgment is pervasive across medical specialties. Even within the same medical field, variations exist in how physicians assess and make decisions. Additionally, differences in clinical judgment may emerge when specialists from distinct disciplines collaborate. This can occur when a physician narrows their focus to a particular area of expertise and overlooks the broader clinical context [18].

Engaging with Consultants

When a challenging physician seeks consultation but subsequently disregards the consultant's recommendations, it may signal a persistent pattern of behaviour. This pattern may suggest that the physician (1) places a lower value on and lacks trust in the expertise of consultants when compared to their own clinical judgment, and/or (2) utilises consultations primarily as a means to address legal concerns, rather than actively aiming to enhance the quality of patient care. These interactions with challenging colleagues can also contribute to the burnout experienced by consultants [19].

Addressing "Challenging" or "Problematic" Colleagues

It is an unequivocal obligation for fellow medical professionals to report doctors who display evident signs of psychosis or addiction. Such instances require clear and unambiguous action. Medical practitioners are both morally and legally bound to report colleagues engaged in overtly unlawful activities, including but not limited to inappropriate relationships with patients and/or medical trainees [20].

Dealing with Physicians with Personality Disturbances

To address physicians with personality disturbances, starting with communication awareness through training modules is crucial. Understanding complex communication issues among medical professionals involves exploring group dynamics theories. When dealing with physicians exhibiting personality disorders, strict rules and boundaries are necessary, with the option of therapy or disciplinary actions if initial interventions fail. Programs involving external psychiatrists have been proposed for rehabilitating impaired physicians. Success in managing physicians with psychosis or addiction hinges on their acknowledgment of the need for psychiatric treatment for reinstatement. Handling the most challenging physicians, involved in unethical or criminal behaviour, poses complex challenges, often resulting in the late-stage diagnosis of severe personality disorders by forensic psychiatrists [15, 19].

Narcissism and arrogance in physicians can lead to a belief that they know better than their colleagues, disrupting medical organisations. Upholding values like intellectual humility and respect, is crucial in clinical practice.

Achievement and professional success can foster arrogance and a lack of respect for differing positions. Some colleagues lack these values. Narcissism and arrogance in physicians can lead to a belief that they know better than their colleagues, disrupting medical organisations. Upholding values like intellectual humility and respect, is crucial in clinical practice.

Achievement and professional success can foster arrogance and a lack of respect for differing positions. Some colleagues lack these values.

It is recommended to address "disruptive doctors" by emphasising "empathy". Those lacking empathy may struggle in patient-centric specialties but excel in procedure-focused areas. Education modules of professionalism, communication, empathy, and managing conflict have been described by some authorities [15, 16, 21].

References

1. de Leon J, Wise TN, Balon R, Fava GA. Dealing with difficult medical colleagues. Psychother Psychosom. 2018;87(1):5–11.
2. Boisaubin EV, Levine RE. Identifying and assisting the impaired physician. Am J Med Sci. 2001;322:31–6.
3. Morris JM, Clarke C. Mandatory reporting of impaired medical practitioners: protecting patients, supporting practitioners. Intern Med J. 2014;44:1165–9.
4. Reynolds NT. Disruptive physician behavior: use and misuse of the label. J Med Regul. 2012;98:8–19.
5. American Medical Association: Disruptive Physicians. https://com-psychiatry-pep.sites.medinfo.ufl.edu/files/2014/06/AMA-Physicians-and-Disruptive-Behavior-Policy.pdf.
6. Goettler CE, Butler TS, Shackleford P, Rotondo MF. Physician behavior: not ready for "Never" land. Am Surg. 2011;77:1600–5.
7. Myers MM. Physician impairment: is it relevant to academic psychiatry? Acad Psychiatry. 2008;32:39–43.
8. Lillis S, Takai N, Francis S. Long-term outcomes of a remedial education program for doctors with clinical performance deficits. J Contin Educ Heal Prof. 2014;34:96–101.
9. Leape LL, Fromson JA. Problem doctors: is there a system-level solution? Ann Intern Med. 2006;144:107–15.
10. Roback HB, Strassberg D, Iannelli RJ, Finlayson AJ, Blanco M, Neufeld R. Problematic physicians: a comparison of personality profiles by offence type. Can J Psychiatr. 2007;52:315–22.
11. American Psychiatric Association. Diagnostic and statistical manual of mental disorders, 3rd ed, rev (DSM-III-R). Washington: American Psychiatric Association; 1987.
12. Gabbard GO. The role of compulsiveness in the normal physician. JAMA. 1985;254:2926–9.
13. Finlayson AJ, Dietrich MS, Neufeld R, Roback H, Martin PR. Restoring professionalism: the physician fitness-for-duty evaluation. Gen Hosp Psychiatry. 2013;35:659–63.
14. Gruppen LD. Humility and respect: core values in medical education. Med Educ. 2014;48:53–8.
15. Baron-Cohen S. The science of evil. On empathy and the origins of cruelty. New York: Basic Books; 2011.
16. Mechanic D. The functions and limitations of trust in the provision of medical care. J Health Polit Policy Law. 1998;23:661–86.
17. Fava GA, Tomba E, Sonino N. Clinimetrics: the science of clinical measurements. Int J Clin Pract. 2012;66:11–5.
18. Wise TN, Berlin RM. Burnout: stresses in consultation-liaison psychiatry. Psychosomatics. 1981;22:744–51.
19. Howe EG. What do we owe medical students and medical colleagues who are impaired? J Clin Ethics. 2016;27:87–98.

20. Cima M, Tonnaer F, Hauser MD. Psychopaths know right from wrong but don't care. Soc Cogn Affect Neurosci. 2010;5:59–67.
21. Nasca TJ, Philibert I, Brigham T, Flynn TC. The new GME accreditation system – rationale and benefits. N Engl J Med. 2012;366:1051–6.

Chapter 30
Doctors, Patients, and Lawyers

The close association between law and medicine has endured for a minimum of the last two centuries. Herman Melville's 1851 literary work, "Moby-Dick," serves as a metaphorical masterpiece from Massachusetts. It symbolises the perspective shared by numerous physicians, both in the past and today, that medical malpractice litigation is akin to the elusive white whale—deemed malevolent, omnipresent, and seemingly everlasting. The relationship between physicians and lawyers was not necessarily more amicable than it is today, mainly due to the presence of medical malpractice litigation.

In the last two centuries, the field of medical jurisprudence, which applies medical knowledge to serve justice, has transformed into legal medicine, encompassing forensic science. The integration of law and medicine has evolved significantly during this period, paralleling changes in medical practice. Health law has a strong connection with medical ethics. Notably, Thomas Percival's 1803 influential text on Medical Ethics, one of the most significant treatises on the subject in the last two centuries, was originally titled "Medical Jurisprudence." A substantial portion of Percival's work delves into "professional duties requiring legal knowledge."

During the early and mid-nineteenth century, the primary focus areas of medical jurisprudence included forensic pathology, which involved determining the cause of death in criminal cases, particularly when poisoning was suspected, and forensic psychiatry, which aimed to establish, for instance, the mental state of a defendant at the time they committed a crime. Some authorities of medical ethics believed that physicians should know enough law to be useful and credible witnesses in court. "A doctor who knows nothing of law, and a lawyer who knows nothing of medicine, are deficient in essential requisites of their respective professions." [1–3].

In the notable case of Slater v. Baker and Stapleton in 1767 England, Slater sought treatment from physician Baker and apothecary Stapleton for a poorly healed broken leg. They attempted a drastic intervention using a "heavy steel device with teeth" to reset the leg, but it yielded unsatisfactory results. Slater sued them, and three surgeons testified against the use of this device. The jury awarded Slater £500 (equivalent to about £60,000 today), and the defendants appealed. The appeals court

S. Abbas, *Medical Ethics*, https://doi.org/10.1007/978-981-96-9199-9_30

upheld the verdict, highlighting that radical medical experiments could constitute malpractice, particularly when conducted without the patient's consent. The court record says: "this was the first experiment made with this new instrument; and although the defendants in general may be as skilful, yet in this particular case they have acted ignorantly and unskilfully, contrary to the known rule and usage of surgeons" [4].

Elwell raised a valid objection to the court's assertion that a physician, simply by conducting a unique experiment, is automatically deemed "guilty of rashness and recklessness." "Suggests a significant presence of criminal intent or imprudent and blameworthy recklessness [that could render the physician] genuinely culpable of a criminal offence.

His perspective was not isolated in that era. It is been noted independently that "between 1845 and 1861, physicians were genuinely alarmed by the surge in malpractice claims." In 1850, a communication to the Massachusetts Medical Society highlighted the "alarmingly frequent" prosecutions for malpractice. The Massachusetts Medical Society proposed the engagement of an impartial physician to assess malpractice threats from disgruntled patients, For many physicians, medical malpractice litigation is akin to the elusive white whale—a persistent danger. Lawyers, in this context, are often perceived as sharks or vultures [5, 6].

Applying legal principles to healthcare, has vastly expanded. The recognition of patients' rights and the broadening of regulatory oversight in medical practices have significantly expanded the field. Landmark judgments, like those from the Nuremberg trial of Nazi doctors, particularly influenced the development of patients' rights, including the doctrine of informed consent [7].

While malpractice continues to be a concern, key legal issues in modern medical practice revolve around the fiduciary nature of the doctor–patient relationship. These encompass

(a) patient rights
(b) patient safety
(c) informed consent
(d) privacy
(e) commercialisation
(f) the regulation of medical research and bio-banking, gene and cell line patenting
(g) the utilisation of genomic information in medical practice,
(h) racial disparities
(i) ensuring equitable access to quality medical care

The increased incidence of litigation led to development of defensive practice of medicine. Indeed, 90% of physicians surveyed in high-liability specialties disclosed engaging in "defensive medicine" due to their apprehension about litigation [8].

Negligence

Patients often experience significant harm due to medical interventions, with many injuries attributed to below-standard care. Law denotes a collection of regulations enforced by a nation's legal system. It comprises common law derived from precedents and statutory law based on parliamentary legislation. Court-ordered common law, rooted in precedent, typically yields to statutory law unless specific circumstances are not covered by statutes. A tort is a civil wrongdoing addressed by common law or statutory law, and medical negligence falls under this category, with compensatory damages (monetary compensation) being the usual remedy [9].

The notions of adverse events and negligence are directly derived from the principles of tort law, encompassing medical malpractice. Litigation on negligence should be linked to quality assurance. There has been a consistent rise in malpractice claims against healthcare providers, accompanied by an increase in monetary damages awarded to plaintiffs. Reducing claims needs to be addressed mainly by improving the delivered care and promoting quality-of-care initiatives. Advocates for tort reform contend that the current malpractice litigation system is inefficient in compensating patients harmed by medical practices and deterring poor-quality care that may lead to injuries. On the other hand, some defend the role of tort litigation. These debates are likely to persist even as claim rates start to decline [10].

A typical example is: "A 60 years old man experienced rectal bleeding. Despite the patient's continued symptoms, the physician only conducted a limited, negative sigmoidoscopy and reassured the patient. A year later, following a significant weight loss of 10 kg, he was admitted to the hospital and diagnosed with colon cancer with liver metastases. Upon reviewing his medical record, physicians concluded that appropriate diagnostic measures could have identified the cancer at an earlier, treatable stage. The advanced disease was attributed to substandard medical care, and the event was deemed adverse and a result of negligence."

Negligence, as a tort, has evolved into the most significant tort, now forming the basis of liability in nearly every human undertaking. In recent decades, it has transitioned from primarily addressing physical injury and property damage to encompassing economic loss and psychiatric diseases. Establishing a predictable and coherent set of principles to achieve justice and minimise negative repercussions to the community has proven challenging. Despite this, there are some general approaches to building a case of medical negligence [11]. It involves the following steps:

1. Establishing a duty of care; This duty is inherent in the doctor–patient relationship.
2. Breach of duty: This involves comparing the healthcare provider's actions to what a reasonably other practitioner would have done.
3. Establishing causation, and the scope of liability: It needs to be established that the breach of duty directly caused the patient's injuries or harm. This is often a critical element, requiring a clear connection between the healthcare provider's actions and the resulting harm.

4. Consideration of defences: Defendants may employ various defences to counter the allegations brought against them. Two commonly used defences are: Contributory Negligence: This defence suggests that the plaintiff's own actions or negligence caused their injuries. If this is the case, they cannot recover damages. New Intervening Events: This defence asserts that unforeseen events occurred. These events, often called intervening or superseding events, may include a patient's non-compliance with post-treatment instructions or the occurrence of unrelated medical complications. If the defence can prove that these events were the primary cause of the harm, the defendant may be liable less.
5. It's important to note that the effectiveness of these defences can vary depending on jurisdiction and the specific circumstances of the case. Additionally, legal arguments and evidentiary support play crucial roles in determining the success of these defences in countering medical negligence claims.
6. Damages and compensation: The plaintiff must demonstrate that they suffered actual harm or damages as a result of the healthcare provider's negligence. This can include physical injuries, emotional distress, financial loss, or other measurable harm. Medical negligence cases often involve healthcare professionals providing expert opinions on the standard of care, the breach of that standard, causation, and resulting damages. Medical records, expert reports, and other evidence are crucial [11].

In medical negligence cases, "Understanding the distinction between blameworthy behaviour and inevitable human errors and appreciating the systemic factors that underlie most failures in complex systems are essential. It is important to meet society's needs to blame and exact retribution when appropriate. However, this should not be a pre-requisite for compensation …" [12].

Common Medical Errors of Negligence

Avoidance

Ensure compassionate care if a major event happens, including making rounds in the presence of relatives after a bad outcome, to convey understanding and support. Maintain eye contact to reassure patients and relatives.

Failure to Communicate

Communicate diagnosis, treatment, and medication plans clearly. Confirm patient understanding by having them explain the information back. This fosters proper adherence and demonstrates genuine care toward the patient.

Miss Diagnosis

Making diagnosis challenging. Recognise and adapt to the developing technology and review that in light of patients concern, which doctors tend to rely on extensively which at times can lead to diagnostic error.

Failure to Identify Complications

Complications are very common in procedural intervention, any complication could be addressed easily when picked early.

Inadequate Follow-Up

Establish robust follow-up systems to track test results and patient compliance.

Not Listening to Patients Concern

Invest adequate time to build trust in allowing patients to fully express their concerns. The physician's ability to demonstrate concern, empathy, and likability is directly related to the time spent with the patient. Increased quality time reduces the likelihood of legal action.

Prescribing Errors

Before prescribing medications, be aware of all drugs the patient is taking. Reinforce the importance of proper medication adherence and prompt communication if any concerns arise. Utilise electronic prescribing to minimise errors and work collaboratively with hospital pharmacists to prevent drug interactions [13, 14].

Other issues in relation to informed consent and rigorous documentation are covered elsewhere.

Certain nations have implemented a no-fault medical compensation scheme, simultaneously abandoning their previous medical negligence-based compensation systems. Under this system, damages are funded by an insurance pool, while an independent body oversees the standard of care, effectively separating compensation from deterrence [15].

Patients affected by negligent medical care may choose to file a lawsuit or may not, while paradoxically, patients who have received damages may not have been subjected to a doctor's negligent care. The concerning data indicates that, in 3% of claims, there were no verifiable medical injuries, and 37% did not involve errors. Logically, the majority of claims involving injuries due to errors did indeed have medical injuries or errors (73%). However, the "reassuring data" reveals that most claims not associated with errors (72%) or injuries (84%) did not result in compensation [16].

Doctors can proactively mitigate the risk of medical litigation and enhance the overall quality of patient care. To minimise the risk of medical litigation for doctors, several strategies can be implemented:

1. Communication: Establish clear and open communication with patients. Explain their diagnosis, treatment options, and risks. Address questions promptly.
2. Consent: Informed consent is required for medical procedures. Clear risks, benefits, and alternatives must be explained. Documented.
3. Documentation: Maintain accurate and comprehensive medical records. Document patient interactions, diagnoses, treatment plans, and informed consent discussions. Documented records are valuable in court.
4. Best Practices: Adhere to evidence-based medical practices and guidelines. Stay informed about best practices in your field.
5. Collaboration: Consult with other healthcare professionals when necessary.
6. Continuous Education: Engage in professional development and education to enhance patient care.
7. Establish Policies and Protocols: Develop and implement clear policies and protocols in your medical practice.
8. Effective Risk Management: Identify risks, implement preventive measures, and develop protocols to address emerging issues.
9. Compassion: Deliver compassionate, patient-centred care to address patient concerns promptly [16, 17].
10. Professional Liability Insurance: Ensure that you have adequate professional liability insurance coverage.

The Impact on Doctors Health

There the to be profound psychological effects of a malpractice claim on doctors, indicating that affected physicians are more prone to altering their care practices, often resorting to defensive medicine measures with risk of anxiety and depression, frustration, anger, insomnia, and exacerbation of physical illness. Physicians undergoing a formal disciplinary process experienced heightened levels of depression, anxiety, and contemplation of self-harm. Doctors who are going through litigation undergo serious impairment of performance during the litigation process, with more negative attitudes toward their work and social and patient' relations, many of them described the experience as the most traumatic in their lives, with increasing risk of suicide [18, 19].

Despite research and organisational insights, regulatory authorities have shown limited formal acknowledgment of the substantial impact that complaints can have on practitioners and the imperative to mitigate this impact [20]. Medical defence organisations should play a crucial role in supporting their members by providing education about the legal process and ensuring a comprehensive understanding of how medico-legal issues can impact both personal and professional aspects of their lives [21].

Enhancing the promptness of handling complaints and ensuring equitable time frames for practitioners to respond to regulator requests would significantly enhance practitioners' experiences within the regulatory process and bolster public confidence in the regulator. Regulators should take the next step by officially recognising the substantial impact regulatory processes can impose on practitioners. They must persist in implementing enhancements to ensure fairness, transparency, and timeliness, aiming to reduce the potential harm to those under regulation [21].

References

1. Percival T. Medical ethics. Manchester: S. Russell; 1803. p. 7.
2. Beauchamp TL, Childress JF. Principles of biomedical ethics. 5th ed. New York: Oxford University Press; 2001. p. 31.
3. Channing W. A medico-legal treatise on malpractice and medical evidence—a review. Boston Med Surg J. 1860;62:233-41,259-65,300-7.
4. Slater v. Baker and Stapleton, C.B. Eng. Rptr. 860 (Michelmas Term, 8 Geo III, 1767).
5. Elwell JJ. A medico-legal treatise on malpractice and medical evidence: comprising the elements of medical jurisprudence. New York: John S. Voorhies; 2013.
6. Mehlman MJ. The shame of medical malpractice. J Leg Med. 2006;27:17–32.
7. Annas GJ, Grodin MA. The Nazi doctors and the Nuremberg code: human rights in human experimentation. New York: Oxford University Press; 1992.
8. Studdert DM, Mello MM, Sage WM, et al. Defensive medicine among high-risk specialist physicians in a volatile malpractice environment. JAMA. 2005;293(21):2609–17.
9. Brennan TA, Leape LL, Laird NM, et al. Incidence of adverse events and neg-ligence in hospitalized patients: results of the Harvard medical practice study I. N Engl J Med. 1991;324(6):370–6.
10. Siegel DR. An overview of medical malpractice legislation. N Y State J Med. 1986;86:377–91.
11. AIHW, Australia's Medical Indemnity Claims 2012–13, Australian Institute of Health and Welfare, Canberra. 2014.
12. Runciman WB, Merry AF, Tito F. Error, blame, and the law in health care – an antipodean perspective. Ann Intern Med. 2003;138(12):974–9.
13. Hagihara A, Tarumi K. Association between physicians' communicative behaviors and judges' decisions in lawsuits on negligent care. Health Policy. 2007;83 213–22.
14. Raveesh BN, Nayak RB, Kumbar SF. Preventing medico-legal issues in clinical practice. Ann Indian Acad Neurol. 2016;19(Suppl 1):S15–20. https://doi.org/10.4103/0972-2327.192886. PMID: 27891020; PMCID: PMC5109754.
15. OECD. Medical malpractice. OECD; 2006.

16. Studdert DM, Mello MM, Gawande AA, et al. Claims, errors, and compensation payments in medical malpractice litigation. N Engl J Med. 2006;354(19):2024–33.
17. Sappideen C. Medical teams and the standard of care in negligence. J Law Med. 2015;23(1):69–82.
18. Nash L, Daly M, Van Ekert E, Kelly P. The medico-legal environment and how medico-legal matters impact the doctor. In: Figley C, Huggard P, Rees C, editors. First do no self-harm: understanding and promoting physician stress resilience. New York: Oxford University Press; 2013.
19. Bourne T, Wynants L, Peters M, et al. The impact of complaints procedures on the welfare, health and clinical practice of 7962 doctors in the UK: a cross- sectional survey. BMJ Open. 2015;4:e006687.
20. Sparrow M. The art of harm reduction. What is a 'risk-based regulator' and would you like to be one? In: Paper presented at 11th international conference on medical regulation. London: International Conference on Medical Regulation; 2014.
21. Australian Health Practitioner Regulation Agency. Annual report 2013/2014. Canberra: AHPRA, 2014. Haysom G. Complaint consequences. MJA Insight 2013: 9 December. Available at www.mja.com.au/insight/2013/47/georgie-haysom-complaint-consequences.

Chapter 31
Ethics in Human Genomic Medicine

The field and term "genetics" originated in the early twentieth century. The term "new" genetics signifies the significant advancements in genetic understanding resulting from the increased knowledge of the biochemical basis in deoxyribonucleic acid (DNA). In the late 1980s, when the proposal for substantial funding for the Human Genome Project was introduced in the United States, Dr. James Watson, the project's initial director, recommended allocating 5% of the funding to investigate the "ethical, social, and legal implications" (ELSI) of human genetics.

Some ethical problems cannot be tested in real life, so moral scientist designed thought experiment. Thought experiments exist along a spectrum of diverse experiments, offering a conduit to access a rich repository of "instinctive knowledge" acquired from past experiences. Imagine being a physician attending to a young patient with a family history of a fatal heritable disease characterised by significant suffering, typically surfacing in late middle life. No therapy exists for this condition, and the patient is unaware of its hereditary nature, holding a 50% chance of carrying the dominant gene. The speed of finding new genetic information is astonishing which will provide large-scale genetic testing and gene therapy. For example, the testing of nucleotide polymorphism will enable doctors to identify in advance which patient would respond to certain medications. Genetic testing requires fully informed consent so the patient understands and agrees to the potential issues that could arise from the test. These issues can be psychological, social, and issues related to confidentiality of the acquired genetic data.

A genomic test is available to ascertain the likelihood of developing the disease. The ethical quandary is whether to inform the patient about the prognosis, heritability, and the option of a genomic test for diagnosis [1].

This thought experiment is notably challenging, with the decision to discuss the condition contingent on personal familiarity with the patient and my evaluation of their ability to cope with the ensuing uncertainty. The consideration of whether to discuss testing options also depends on my assessment of potential outcomes. A comparable situation arises in patients with the gene for Huntington's chorea, where knowledge of gene status or symptom onset may lead to suicide. Huntington's

S. Abbas, *Medical Ethics*, https://doi.org/10.1007/978-981-96-9199-9_31

chorea is inherited as an autosomal dominant gene, ensuring the inevitable development of the condition and severe neurological deterioration if the gene is present.

Even if our thought experiment patient chooses not to undergo genomic testing, a lingering sense of potential doom remains. Knowledge of the genomic analysis results would likely influence future decisions, such as those regarding family and career. This clinical ethics dilemma is intricate, and I remain uncertain about presenting all options to such a patient [2, 3].

In October 2018, the United Kingdom's National Health Service (NHS) incorporated whole genome sequencing into standard NHS care, initiating the world's first "Genomic Medicine Service." Other nations, such as France and Canada, are in different phases of developing comparable publicly funded genomic healthcare services, principally for the diagnosis of suspected heritable conditions and for targeting cancer treatments [5].

Advancements in DNA analysis and comprehension carry ethical implications for society, primarily concerning the predictive capacity of DNA, from conception to birth and throughout an individual's life. These implications extend to healthcare, identity establishment, uncovering historical information, genetic manipulation, ownership and control of genetic material and data, as well as cultural perspectives on humanity, race, and the interplay between heredity and nurture. Different techniques for examining hundreds, and eventually millions, of "single nucleotide markers" in a human genome through "SNP chips" now come at a cost below $100, resulting in their widespread utilisation in scientific "genome-wide association studies" over the last two decades. The late 1960s witnessed increasing discussions regarding human cloning, with safety concerns about recombinant DNA and social worries about genetic discrimination arising in the 1970s and early 1980s. The social concerns related to genomics centre around the risks of human genomics being misused, including concerns about privacy loss, genetic discrimination, and the potential for state-enforced eugenics, but we have to think about but in the expectation that the research will bring immense medical benefits. A continuous flow of novel treatments, stemming from enhanced understanding of genomes and their linked proteins, is progressing through research, development, and regulatory approval—albeit not as swiftly as desired, but consistently [4, 5].

Genomics introduces four primary concerns related to identity: forensic identification, personal identity, family identity, and ethnic identity. Any tissue containing DNA can now be tested for distinctive markers, specific sections of the genome that exhibit substantial variability among individuals. These markers can be compared with those obtained from human tissue or secretions and hairs or blood associated with a crime [6].

The current concerns for society at large regarding the forensic utilisation of DNA primarily revolve around the broader aspects of DNA collection and storage for identification purposes, rather than individual cases. One key issue involves the potential clandestine gathering of DNA by law enforcement agencies from suspects. This can occur through various means, including engaging with suspects, such as offering them a drink and obtaining DNA from the discarded container, or collecting DNA from items they have touched, ranging from cigarette butts to eating utensils [7]. The dan data get stored for future criminal investigations.

The first involves their creation. Should samples be accepted only from those who consent or should they be mandatory? If mandatory, what classes of people should be required to provide samples—convicted sex offenders, convicted felons, all those arrested, or the whole population? Litigation on this issue has become increasingly common in the United States, where all states have some form of mandatory DNA repository. Alonzo Jay King Jr. was charged with first and second-degree assault. The Supreme Court heard the case in February 2013, delivering a verdict 4 months later in June 2013. In line with Maryland police protocol and the Maryland DNA Collection Act, a DNA sample was collected from King during his arrest. This sample later matched an unsolved rape case from 2003 [8]. The supreme court maintained that "categorically" and "without exception," "The Fourth Amendment forbids searching a person for evidence of a crime when there is no basis for believing the person is guilty of the crime or is in possession of incriminating evidence" [9]. The case revolves around the matter of consent, as King did not provide consent for a cheek swab, which resulted in his DNA being included in the Maryland DNA database.

Cloning and Personal Identity

The controversy over somatic cell nuclear transfer technology for human cloning raises familiar issues from in vitro fertilisation and advanced reproductive technologies. The unique concern with cloning revolves around human identity, questioning whether an individual with the same genome as another would be, in essence, a copy of that person. The application of new methods has indeed generated seemingly viable human embryos and embryonic stem cells from these cloned embryos. This development has, to some degree, reignited concerns about the potential birth of human clones.

Familial Identity

Affordable genomic analysis enables the use of DNA to confirm or disprove close family connections. This type of family analysis, utilising inexpensive SNP chips and examining variations on the Y chromosome (exclusive to men and inherited from father to son) or mitochondrial DNA (present in both men and women but inherited solely from the mother), has spurred the expansion of a consumer genetic genealogy sector. It could reused to track and identify unknown parents particularly when the mother is trying to identify the genetic father for child support and cases of adoption. The ethical considerations associated with utilising DNA for confirming or disproving family connections can differ, frequently contingent upon the consent of the identified or potentially estranged family members involved. Ethnicities or nations frequently not only have common cultures but also share a significant degree of shared ancestry [10].

Selection

Prenatal testing has been employed for several decades to prevent severe genetic diseases. Initial initiatives involved screening for conditions such as thalaseamia sickle cell anaemia and Tay-Sachs disease. Prospective parents can use this information to make decisions about marriage, having children, or undergoing prenatal testing. Carrier testing, with informed consent, has become more widespread and less controversial, particularly with the availability of commercial tests covering over a hundred genetic disease traits at affordable prices. Also prenatal testing for trisomy 21 by taking a sample of the pregnant woman blood. Foetal genetic testing has sparked controversy, with opponents condemning it for its association with abortion, viewed by some as an act of murder. Advocates for individuals with disabilities express particular concern about such testing, especially when it results in subsequent abortions. Some argue that this belief suggests that individuals with those genetic conditions are deemed to have lives not worth living. In the United States, abortion is legally permissible for any reason until the foetus is viable outside the womb, leading to limited discussions about outlawing abortion.

An alternative approach altering discussions on prenatal genetic testing is "preimplantation genetic diagnosis" (PGD), allowing testing of a young embryo before implantation. This procedure is exclusive to in vitro fertilisation. A single cell is detached and its DNA tested, enabling parents to decide whether to implant that embryo or, more practically, which tested embryo to choose. Moreover, in the coming decades, the requirement for egg harvest, the costliest, least pleasant, and riskiest element of in vitro fertilisation, could be circumvented by utilising skin or other cells from a woman to generate new eggs [11].

The concept of employing genetic testing to choose "enhanced" genetic traits for offspring has prompted numerous concerns. Concerns include the fear that allowing parents to select or believe they can select their children's traits may infringe upon the children's right to an open future not dictated by their parents. There are also worries about economic disparities, as the wealthy could potentially purchase genetic advantages for their offspring, while those conceiving traditionally may be denied such opportunities. Additionally, there is a concern that parental selection could lead to a homogenisation of the human gene pool if parents consistently choose children with similar traits. Sex selection is a form of "genetic enhancement," achievable through sonography or genetic testing. In certain countries, prenatal sex selection through abortion is prevalent, with female foetuses aborted more frequently than males. This practice is poised to create significant imbalances in the sex ratio, potentially leading to widespread social consequences [12].

Genetic testing extends beyond birth, aiding in the diagnosis of diseases or the prediction of future health risks. As with all medical interventions. It can provide information that can lead to a medical intervention, and help the patient make life plans. However, the test results can lead to psychological problems for patients and affect their social relations, their employment, and health insurance discrimination. The advantages of testing for children might be delayed until they reach adulthood and can independently make informed decisions about testing unless the test can lead to useful early intervention such as phenylketonuria. These concerns become especially worrisome when considering tests for children, particularly if the presently obligatory neonatal genetic testing is substituted with whole genome sequencing, which could lead to finding other genetic variations [13, 14].

There has been significant apprehension regarding the potential misuse of genetic tests for discriminating against individuals based on genetically anticipated susceptibilities, particularly with health insurance.

In 2008, the United States enacted the Genetic Information Non-Discrimination Act, which largely prohibited the utilisation of genetic information in both employment and health insurance [15].

Gene Therapy

Somatic cell gene therapy seeks to cure a disease exclusively within the patient, without affecting the patient's descendants. Originally, it was envisioned as introducing a properly functioning copy of a gene into an individual with a genetic disease caused by inheriting only malfunctioning gene copies. The genetic components of somatic cell gene therapy have been mostly non-controversial. Essentially, gene therapy is just another drug delivery system. Germ line gene therapy has been much more controversial. it involves the introduction of "normal" human genes into the eggs or sperm, or into the fertilised egg or early embryo of the offspring. The objective is to alter the genetic inheritance of the child, either to prevent a genetic disease or to introduce an "enhancing" genetic variation. Human germline gene therapy in its traditional sense has not been attempted; there has been an informal moratorium in the scientific community on conducting such experiments in humans, based on the concern that gene alteration could have unforeseeable consequences for future generations [16].

Ensuring the safety of generating new genes, and consequently, new proteins or genomes, leading to new organisms, is an evident concern. This became particularly relevant after the discovery of the CRISPR DNA editing which can alter any given gene, it also can be used to turn the gene on or off without alterations. This technology has the potential to transform medicine to enable not only treatment but also prevention of some diseases, and altering certain characteristics in children. We generally think human genome editing for reproductive purposes should not be allowed. There has been an international effort led by United States and China to coordinate regulations that govern the application of genome editing.

The creation of new genes is now possible. This raises questions about who owns genetic material and who should have access to it. The more profound question revolves around whether humanity should assume the role of "playing God" by deliberately creating such novel entities. Gene patenting raises moral and cultural questions about whether it is ethically appropriate to claim ownership over parts of the human genome, which is a shared and fundamental aspect of humanity. Enhancement of certain human characteristics, which is technically possible, is generally prohibited because it could lead to advancing some people at the expense of others, also it raises problems about equity if the rich can afford the enhancement therapy which will disadvantage the poor.

Another concern about gremlin DNA editing is the lack of consent because the patient affected by the editing is an embryo.

It could commodify and commercialise aspects of human existence. Also, it may contribute to global health disparities, as access to patented genetic technologies may be limited in certain regions, affecting healthcare equity. Some argue that gene patents can stifle innovation and research by restricting the ability of scientists and researchers to study and develop therapies based on patented genes [15, 16].

Stem Cell Therapy Research

While it is prohibited by the European Union, other countries have approved the research. An important aspect of the debate revolves around the necessity of using embryos for stem cell therapy research, with the prevailing scientific opinion supporting its requirement. If this viewpoint is accurate, the central dilemma becomes whether the potential advancement of a new realm in regenerative medicine outweighs ethical concerns related to experimenting on or terminating human embryos. According to some, it is immoral because it terminates lives like abortion and is often articulated as "respect for human life" or the sanctity of life, "life" is "clearly not referring to the pure and simple fact of biological existence." The objection could be raised on the basis that the embryos being experimented upon would not exist if it were not for scientific intervention or creation. In other words, the argument acknowledges the artificial or created nature of the embryos and anticipates that someone might raise an objection based on this premise. There is an ongoing debate that revolves around the meaning of life which got to be beyond biological existence [17, 18].

References

1. Cook-Deegan RM. The gene wars: science, politics, and the human genome. New York: Norton; 1994.

2. Schoenfeld M, Myers RH, Cupples LA, et al. Increased rate of suicide among patients with Huntington's disease. J Neurol Neurosurg Psychiatry. 1984;47:1283–128.
3. Warburton N. A little history of philosophy. New Haven: Yale University Press; 2011. p. 222–33.
4. Delaney SK, Hultner ML, Jacob HJ, Ledbetter DH, McCarthy JJ, Ball M, et al. Toward clinical genomics in everyday medicine: perspectives and recommendations. Expert Rev Mol Diagn. 2016;16:521–32.
5. Annas GJ, Glantz LH, Roche PA. The genetic privacy act and commentary. Boston: Boston University School of Health; 1995.
6. National Research Council. DNA technology in forensic science. Washington, DC: National Academy Press; 1992.
7. National Research Council. DNA technology in forensic science: an update. Washington, DC: National Academy Press; 1996.
8. Maryland v. King, 133 S.Ct. 1958, 2013.
9. King, 569 U.S. at 466 (Scalia, J., dissenting).
10. Greely HT, Riordan DP, Garrison NA, Mountain JL. Family ties: the use of DNA offender databases to catch offenders' kin. J Law Med Ethics. 2006;34:248–62.
11. Greely HT. Get ready for the flood of fetal gene screening. Nature. 2011;469:289–91. Hvistendahl M. Unnatural selection: choosing boys over girls, and the consequences of a world full of men. New York: Public Affairs. 2011.
12. Parens E. Enhancing human traits: ethical and social implications. Washington, DC: Georgetown University Press; 1998.
13. Institute of Medicine, U.S. National Academy of Sciences. Assessing genetic risks: implications for health and social policy. Washington, DC: National Academy Press; 1993.
14. Ormond KE, Wheeler MT, Hudgins L, Klein TE, Butte AJ, Altman RB, Ashley EA, Greely HT. Challenges in the clinical application of whole- genome sequencing. Lancet. 2010;375:1749–51.
15. Greely HT. Genotype discrimination. Univ Pa Law Rev. 2001;149:1483–505.
16. Nelson R. Gene therapy, ethics, germ cell gene transfer. In: Murray TH, Mehlman MJ, editors. Encyclopedia of ethical, legal, and policy issues in biotechnology. New York: Wiley; 2000.
17. Marcel G. Life and the sacred in tragic wisdom and beyond. Evanston: Northwestern University Press; 1973. p. 104–19.
18. Boyd KM. Medical ethics: principles, persons, and perspectives: from controversy to conversation. J Med Ethics. 2005;31:481–6.

Chapter 32
Care Givers and Patients with Drug Dependence

Doctors often have ethical issues in managing intoxication and withdrawal from diverse substances (including opioids, sedative-hypnotics, stimulants, and hallucinogens). Encountering drug-dependent patients is an inevitable aspect of contemporary medical practice. Individuals struggling with substance abuse cut across diverse demographics, encompassing various ages, genders, ethnicities, and socioeconomic backgrounds. Providing extended care for chemical dependency is a challenging and occasionally frustrating endeavour, yet it can also be a gratifying journey. The doctor must exercise heightened caution when interacting with patients experiencing withdrawal. Individuals in this state frequently express complaints of pain or anxiety, creating a perceived necessity for prescribing opiates or benzodiazepines.

The American Psychiatric Association's Diagnostic and Statistical Manual characterises opioid use disorder as a problematic pattern involving prescription and/or illicit opioid medication use, resulting in significant clinical impairment or distress. Individuals with opioid use disorder experience poorer overall health and more adverse health service outcomes. This includes higher rates of morbidity, mortality, HIV, and HCV transmission. Given the alarming rate of fatal opioid overdoses, prominent scientific and professional bodies have declared opioid use disorder a public health emergency in the United States. Substance use disorders (SUD), also known as addictions or drug abuse, are persistent, recurring conditions that often coexist with other physical and mental health conditions, as well as intricate social backgrounds. Certain patients, particularly those using crystal meth, may exhibit acute intoxication leading to psychotic symptoms and extreme violence. This poses risks to staff, the patient, and others in the vicinity [1].

Severe skin and heart infections arising from unsafe injection practices are particularly important. These infections are managed with intravenous antibiotics, often administered through a central line. However, central lines pose a risk, as they offer convenient access for the injection of illicit drugs, increasing the risk of overdose. Unsafe practices with central lines can also contribute to the development or worsening of infections. The combination of severe infection, and the very intervention to treat it could lead to worsening addiction and the risk of overdose, poses a

S. Abbas, *Medical Ethics*, https://doi.org/10.1007/978-981-96-9199-9_32

dilemma for physicians as the intervention can lead to worse outcomes if the patient is discharged for home administration of long-term antibiotics.

Considerations in Providing Care for Individuals Using Drugs may include ethical responsibilities on the healthcare providers, such as harm reduction and how do we address and mitigate the violence associated with the drug abuse. What level of intensity is appropriate for treating the consequences (infections) of problematic drug use? Is it advisable to demand abstinence from substance use during treatment for individuals with substance use disorders? When it comes to individuals who inject drugs, should central lines be administered, and if so, should safe injection practices be taught, How can the healthcare system effectively manage the resource demands of providing adequate care for individuals undergoing substance use withdrawal [2].

It is imperative for doctors to recognise a patient with substance abuse, particularly if the patient is forthcoming and requesting help to discontinue abuse. In such a situation the doctor will need to refer the patient to drug and alcohol service to start the appropriate treatment plan. In this case, the CAGE questionnaire, initially designed for alcohol use screening, has been adapted for drug use screening, referred to as the CAGE-AID questionnaire. "*C*, Have you ever tried to cut down on your alcohol or drug use? *A*, Do you get annoyed when people comment about your drinking or drug use? *G*, Do you feel guilty about things you have done while drinking or using drugs? *E*, Do you need an eye-opener to get started in the morning" [3].

Certain clues for identifying such patients are violent toxic behaviour, frequent change of job, repeated injuries, marital problems, and driving while intoxicated. Patients experiencing sexual dysfunction symptoms should undergo an assessment to explore potential drug abuse as a potential contributing factor. Patients with needle signs in the arms along the main veins. Inhaling or snorting cocaine may lead to respiratory issues (such as pneumo-mediastinum), as well as nasal mucosa atrophy and perforation of the nasal septum. All patients with hepatitis, HIV, or endocarditis are likely to use injectable drugs. In suspected cases, a urine sample should be obtained for drug screening. The most reliable evidence for long-term drug use involves a thorough history and a urine toxicology screen, the doctors must be inquisitively curious but not accusative. Patient response in this situation will either be emphatic denial or they will feel relieved that they don't have to hide the habit and help is available [4].

Distinguishing substance abuse lies in patients prescribed addictive drugs for chronic conditions, like long-term pain management is challenging. While these patients may experience physical dependence, they might not fulfil the behavioural criteria for drug addiction. Patients who take drugs for pleasure want more soon after a therapeutic level is reached. The patient who requests new prescriptions repeatedly may have a substance abuse disorder. Patients who use prescription drugs might get multiple prescriptions from different doctors. Check with the pharmacy to see if there is drug abuse going on that the pharmacy did not find. Some pharmacists will contact the doctors about the prescriptions coming from different places. Methadone is commonly employed for withdrawal from illegal opioids. However, obtaining a special s Drug Enforcement Administration license is necessary to prescribe methadone for withdrawal or long-term treatment of drug dependence [5].

Many substance-abusing individuals acknowledge the risks of drug use, especially after experiencing acute toxicity or withdrawal. Despite this awareness, they remain drawn to addictive behaviour for various reasons, creating a state of ambivalence, which is a normal component of psychological struggles about changing behaviour from drug abuse and seeking treatment, and remaining abstinent. Some patients, grappling with denial, conceal their substance abuse from others, rationalizing, or minimising its consequences. Recognising drug addiction, a physician's role is to assist patients in resolving ambivalence and denial, facilitating their decision to quit drug use and initiate the path toward change. The doctor needs to demonstrate empathy, involving an understanding of the patient's perspectives without passing judgment, criticising, or blaming. Confrontational approaches are linked to treatment failure, but sometimes careful confrontation could help to overcome ambivalence. The primary obstacles to effective recovery often revolve around accessing treatment. A primary care practitioner can play a crucial role by facilitating access to suitable counselling facilities and other long-term substance abuse treatment facilities. Physicians should be acquainted with local substance abuse treatment programs available for patient referrals [6].

Doctors should engage patients actively in the decision-making process, encouraging personal choice while emphasising accountability. The practitioner's role is to keep motivating the patient to pursue recovery from addictive behaviour. Relapse is very frequent in such patients, in that case, the treatment should be intensified, and these relapses should be used as learning experiences to avoid losing hope. Motivational interviewing can be integrated into a conceptual framework called brief intervention, which is employed in the early treatment of addiction [5, 6].

Obstacles to accessing quality treatment and the recovery process are intricate, arising from a toxic interplay of social and clinical factors, such as cost, limited availability, consultation style, and the stigma associated with seeking help for Substance Use Disorders (SUDs), which often leads to feelings of shame [7].

The following steps are advised: FRAME

1. Feedback: feedback entails raising the patient's awareness of both current and potential adverse consequences of addictive behaviour.
2. Responsibility: promotes individual freedom, fosters accountability for one's choices, and allows the patient to actively engage in the treatment process.
3. Advice: about the long-term consequences of abuse
4. Menu: Involves presenting various options to enable patients to choose strategies that align with their specific needs and circumstances to promote their personal freedom
5. Empathy: entails listening and providing responses that elucidate and enhance the patient's experiences and meanings without imposing the physician's values. It should be done in a way to prevent alienation of patients. Although there is ongoing debate about the nature of empathy, there is a consensus that it should not be limited to mimicking the experiences of others or confused with emotional

contagion or sympathy. The essence of empathy lies in understanding another person's situated psychological states while maintaining clear self-other differentiation. We tend to empathise most easily with those closest to us and less effectively with experiences we do not comprehend.
6. Self-efficacy: Involves fostering patients' confidence in their ability to achieve specific tasks, often by setting simple, attainable early goals that boost self-confidence during recovery.

Person-centred care and supportive relationships should be built between patients and care-givers; guided by both practical and ethical considerations. This type of care prioritises understanding the values and preferences of service users. Ethical drivers emphasise safeguarding the values and rights of individuals. This should be the approach even in the context of concerns about impaired decision-making associated with Substance Use Disorders, in order to promote autonomy and associated with self-determination and independence [8].

It is crucial here to emphasise the important role of empathy in the recovery process. Empathising or understanding the experience of individuals who may intermittently fail to show the same respect poses a substantial moral challenge, particularly for significant others. This challenge is noteworthy as families and significant others are recognised to play a crucial role in the recovery process [9].

The process of decision-making in testing drug abuse is a typical example of relational autonomy. Viewing autonomy solely as individual independence or isolation. Relational autonomy recognises that patients are embedded within various relationships, including family, community, and healthcare–provider interactions. Decisions are shaped not only by individual preferences but also by the dynamics of these relationships. Healthcare professionals engage with patients in a way that respects and considers the patient's values, preferences, and the impact of their decisions on their relationships and social context.

Relational autonomy challenges a purely individualistic understanding of autonomy and encourages a more nuanced and context-dependent approach, recognising the importance of shared decision-making and collaboration. It underscores the idea that autonomy is not exercised in isolation but within a web of relationships and social influences, autonomy can simply be defined as as allowing 'others the freedom to choose their own destiny' [10].

Substance abuse disorders are one of the most stigmatised health conditions as reflected in the attitudes of both the general public and healthcare professionals. In recent times, despite the negative consequences linked to stigma, ethical discussions have arisen, exploring and disputing assertions that stigma plays a beneficial role in managing chronic health conditions associated with behaviour [11].

The research underscores the significance of implementing positive measures to reduce stigma. These measures include education, supporting healthcare providers in engaging with individuals facing stigmatised conditions, direct contact with stigmatised groups/individuals, empowering the stigmatised through a person-centred approach, questioning unconscious biases, and engaging in advocacy and protest [12].

Individuals with substance use disorders may deviate from societal norms, leading to a sense of estrangement from both family and friends, particularly in small rural communities. The interventions most successful in diminishing stigma are those that enhance interaction between the affected group and the broader population. Increased personal connections with individuals experiencing mental illness or addiction decrease the likelihood of moralising, stigmatising, and discriminating against them. Crucial to various approaches for diminishing stigma is the incorporation of strategies to cultivate positive attitudes towards stigmatised conditions. This involves fostering hope and instilling the belief that recovery is achievable. In the context of building an affirmative recovery culture, the emphasis on self-determination and individual choice is considered fundamental. This means recognising and respecting the autonomy of individuals in their recovery journey. In the realm of recovery, it implies that individuals should have the freedom to decide on the path and strategies that best suit their needs. By placing self-determination and individual choice at the crux of the recovery culture, the approach acknowledges that there is no one-size-fits-all solution to addiction and that each person's journey is unique. It encourages a person-centred perspective, where the individual actively participates in decision-making processes related to their treatment, support, and lifestyle changes. This approach fosters empowerment, allowing individuals to take ownership of their recovery and promoting a culture that respects and values their personal agency in the healing process [13].

It is extremely important to keep and confidentiality of the drug-abusing patients unless there is a threat to others. To combat stigma, health system policies should mandate respectful communication standards that refrain from using stigmatising language, ensuring the preservation of patients' dignity with substance use disorders.

The principle of fidelity underscores the importance of truthfulness and commitment to promises in substance abuse counselling. When a counsellor engages with a client, an implicit contract is established, assuming the counsellor's dedication to addressing the client's concerns and maintaining truthful communication. Consent forms, signed by the client, affirm the commitment to confidentiality. However, the counsellor must clarify upfront when certain promises may need to be broken, such as in cases of suicidal or homicidal thoughts or when child abuse is disclosed. The counsellor should be transparent about fidelity limitations to avoid surprises. Additionally, when navigating complex family dynamics or working with clients of questionable competency, the counsellor must stay focused on the primary client's needs and act in accordance with their wishes [13].

Historical patterns reveal that addressing a public health crisis becomes effective when the issue is openly acknowledged. It is ethically imperative for healthcare professionals, insurers, and all those within the healthcare system to extend equal dignity and respect to individuals with Substance Use Disorders as they would to any other patient group. Progress in combating the current opioid crisis requires a shift from blame, shame, and stigma toward an attitude of respect and compassion [14].

It is also important here to highlight the responsibility of prescribing physicians and drug manufacturing firms in the problem of opioid abuse. The pro-opioids for pain management movement, significantly influenced public opinion and subtly shifted perceptions of the medical use of opioids. Consequently, there was a substantial increase in the prescription of opioid analgesics. The issue lies in the proportional correlation between the number of prescriptions and the non-prescribed, diverted use of opioids. The shift from medication to addiction is often subtle and not consciously recognised by the affected individual [15].

One of the primary personal motivations for continuing opioid use is its function as a coping mechanism for life stressors or as a way to self-medicate psychological issues, trauma effects, or emotional pain. Additional, less significant reasons include normalisation (e.g., avoiding discomfort), increased energy, boredom, enhanced sexual intimacy, and self-blame/addictive personality [16].

The opioid epidemic was partially triggered by pharmaceutical companies developing a highly potent opiate analgesic without adequately warning against and in some cases denying, the risk of addiction. A pro-opioids campaign was launched under the false assumption that the use of this medication was entirely free from addiction risk [17].

The behaviour of medical doctors in prescribing opioids should undergo critical scrutiny. When physicians are aware of the addiction risk associated with opioids and still choose to prescribe them, ethical concerns arise. The decision-making process is complex, as the balance between the risk of addiction and the benefit of pain relief requires careful medical and psychological evaluation. Individual differences further complicate the determination of the most suitable treatment. Additionally, the ethical impact extends beyond the medical realm, as the perception of a medication's ethical acceptability is influenced by the doctor's prescription, with far-reaching consequences at both the opinion and action levels, particularly at the subconscious level. This ethical dimension underscores the importance of physicians' responsibility in prescribing medications and the potential societal implications of their choices [18].

It is relevant here to highlight the pertinent ethical issues in drug abusing people infected with HIV.

Within the realms of substance abuse and HIV/AIDS treatment, numerous ethical dilemmas demand specific attention. These issues are explored below in a social and ethical context.

Duty To Treat: The ethical duty to treat takes on heightened significance when addressing disenfranchised populations. Clinicians working with homeless, chronically alcohol-dependent individuals face challenges in securing adequate medical care for HIV-infected clients. Access to essential services, such as dental care, can be elusive. Advocacy within the community becomes crucial for substance abuse treatment professionals. Counsellors and their agencies must project an image of accessibility without imposing restrictions based on individual differences.

Welfare reform and the prominence of managed care accentuate concerns about access, necessitating creative advocacy efforts. Clinicians must strike a balance between ethically sound actions and avoiding inadvertent legal complications, ensuring that duty-to-treat decisions align with agency policies.

Duty To Warn: In the context of HIV-infected substance abusers, unique concerns arise regarding the duty to warn. Beyond the typical obligations related to abuse and threats, providers grapple with clients knowingly transmitting HIV without adequate precautions. Counsellors must tread carefully, considering legal ramifications when taking ethically correct actions. For instance, if a client with HIV fails to inform their partner, the counsellor might face legal liabilities.

Duty-to-warn situations demand a case-by-case examination, with counsellors consulting supervisors and possibly reporting clients to public health departments. The complex nature of knowingly transmitting HIV underscores the need for balancing ethical principles like beneficence, fidelity, and non-maleficence.

End-of-Life Issues: While HIV treatments have significantly lowered AIDS-related mortality, individuals with both HIV and chronic drug use may still face ethical dilemmas related to end-of-life decisions. The advocacy culture among persons with HIV emphasises self-determination, potentially leading clients to decide to discontinue medical interventions.

Clinicians must communicate transparently about confidentiality limitations, especially when clients express intentions related to suicide or ending medical interventions. Understanding jurisdictional laws is vital, and clinicians adhering to professional codes of ethics and institutional standards reduce potential liability concerns.

Dual Relationships: Navigating dual relationships, where providers have both social and professional interactions with clients, presents boundary-related ethical challenges. The potential blurring of lines is more pronounced in rural areas or specific cultural communities.

Although dual relationships should be avoided when possible, clear communication on professional roles and confidentiality is essential when unavoidable. Consistent clarification and frequent checks of client comfort levels help mitigate ethical concerns related to disclosure and trust.

Scarce Resources: Limited resources pose challenges in treating all clients seeking help. Providers must grapple with complex decisions, considering fairness and avoiding bias in resource allocation.

Objective criteria should guide access to services, and a consistent application of these criteria ensures unbiased decisions. Providers may need to adopt review processes to prevent decisions solely based on individual recommendations.

Confidentiality: Confidentiality emerges as a central theme connecting these ethical principles. In the therapeutic relationship, clients must feel their shared information is protected, although managed care requirements and increased data sharing present challenges.

Providers must honestly communicate data reporting requirements to clients and obtain consent for information shared outside the client-provider relationship. Discretion is key in conversations outside the therapeutic relationship, ensuring only relevant information is reported.

In summary, addressing ethical challenges demands a nuanced, case-specific analysis while considering both immediate and long-term consequences of actions.

Balancing legal and ethical responsibilities is essential for providing ethical, effective care [19–21].

Drug Seeking Patient

Drug addiction, a profoundly serious and escalating problem, stands as a paramount public health concern. Among the substances most perilously prone to fostering dependence are opioid derivatives and benzodiazepine sedatives. It can be difficult for Doctors to determine the difference between real medical needs and psychological drug dependence which creates a significant challenge to healthcare providers, both as individuals and institutions. The problem of stigma against drug-dependent patients also contributes to the complexity of this particular health issue that may impact the appropriate care. Formulating the actual diagnosis is a contentious issue, with some experts asserting that the label of "drug seeking" should be entirely avoided due to its potential to engender prejudice, bias, and formidable barriers to compassionate care [22, 23].

The Drug Enforcement Agency, state licensing boards, and at times state judicial bodies have concluded that significant adverse consequences can result, and a healthcare provider may be held responsible for prescribing controlled substances to an individual known to be misusing them [24].

The warning flags listed below are some of the most commonly cited indicators of medication-seeking behavior. There is general agreement on how controlled medication seekers tend to present or can be detected, both in formal chronic pain research and in the less formal assertions made by experts in other healthcare settings and drug enforcement agencies.

A high likelihood of identifying controlled medication-seeking behavior, marked by conspicuous red flags, can be discerned from those exhibiting a more moderate probability, signaled by cautionary yellow flags, through a meticulous review of medical records and astute observations by healthcare providers [25].

Red flags:

Patient frequently visits different providers to obtain controlled medications.
Someone brings a family member to the doctor for a supposed health issue, but then uses the medicine for themselves.
Frequently loses controlled medication by misplacing it or having it stolen.
Has drug-related deterioration in work performance and family relationships.
Concurrently abuses illicit drugs
Steals medical goods, such as prescription pads or syringes
Asking for a certain brand name or dose escalation

Yellow flags:

The patient frequently visits or contacts your facility with requests for refills of the controlled medication or has multiple unsanctioned dose escalations.
Gives an unlikely story for running out of medication, like a family member stole them or the dog ate them or accidentally flushed them down the toilet
Alleged allergy to other no-opioid painkillers
Uses the controlled medication for purposes other than for which it was intended

History of abuse of other substances, such as alcohol or recreational drugs [25].

Saying No is very important if the patient is suspected to be drug-seeking. The approach to prescribing drugs of dependence should be fair and consistent for all patients. Though some patient history factors may signal a higher risk of addiction, anyone can potentially become addicted and care should be exhausted at this point in patients' care.

Practice policy helps them say no. They can state, I do not prescribe these drugs, Our practice avoids prescribing them, or health guidelines recommend against prescribing these, and suggest focusing on other strategies to help with the patient's issue.

Before justifying an ongoing need for a drug of dependence, a full psychosocial assessment should be conducted, previous doctors contacted, and a treatment plan created. Monitoring should include frequent reviews of the patient's function and quality of life, not just symptom resolution. This should be clearly documented. Most patients will have complex issues and need collaborative care, so they should be offered a care plan. Care plans can help patients set goals and identify triggers to prevent drug use.

Doctors should explain the risks and that these drugs are for short-term use until other treatments are effective. Clear time limits should be set from the start, and discussions should focus on the patient's well-being, not judgment. Practices may also use contracts to inform patients about controlled prescribing, boundaries, and treatment risks and benefits. Controlling the prescribing of addictive painkillers should be performed by a specialised pain clinic for patients who need prolonged use of the medications beyond the reasonable time period for the cause [26–28].

References

1. National Institute on Drug Abuse. Opioid Overdose Crisis 2018. https://www.drugabuse.gov/drugs-abuse/opioids/opioid-overdose-crisis.
2. Baldassarri, et al. Debang medical utility, not futility: ethical dilemmas in treating critically ill people who use injectable drugs. J Law Med Ethics. 2018;46(2018):241–51.
3. Brown RL, Rounds LA. Conjoint screening questionnaires for alcohol and other drug abuse: criterion validity in a primary care practice. Wis Med J. 1995:94135–40.
4. Monteiro MG, MLN P, Masur J. The trauma questionnaire for detecting alcohol abuse: limiting factors. Alcohol. 1986:3287–9.
5. Schnoll SH, Finch J. Medical education for pain and addiction: making progress toward answering a need. J Law Med Ethics. 1994:22252–6.
6. Miller WR, Rollnick S. Motivational interviewing: preparing people to change addictive behavior. New York: The Guilford Press; 1991.
7. Institute of Medicine. Improving the quality of healthcare for mental and substance-use conditions: the quality chasm series. Washington, DC: National Academies Press; 2006.
8. Florin D, Dixon J. Public involvement in health care. BMJ. 2004;328(7432):159–61.
9. Miller W, Forcehimes A, Zweben A. Treating addiction: a guide for professionals. New York and London: Guildford Press; 2019.
10. Ryan RM. Psychological needs and the facilitation of integrative processes. J Pers. 1995;63(3):397–427.

11. Bayer R. Stigma and the ethics of public health: not can we but should we. Soc Sci Med. 2008;67(3):463–72.
12. Knaak S, Mantler E, Szeto A. Mental illness-related stigma in healthcare: barriers to access and care and evidence-based solutions. Healthc Manage Forum. 2017;30(2):1116.
13. Corrigan PW, Angell B, Davidson L, et al. From adherence to self-determination: evolution of a treatment paradigm for people with serious mental illnesses. Psychiatr Serv. 2012;63(2):169–73.
14. AMA J Ethics. 2020;22(8):E702–708. https://doi.org/10.1001/amajethics.2020.702.
15. Control CfD. Vital signs: overdoses of prescription opioid pain relievers—United States, 1999–2008. MMWR Morb Mortal Wkly Rep. 2011;60:1487–92.
16. Cicero TJ, Ellis MS. The prescription opioid epidemic: a review of qualitative studies on the progression from initial use to abuse. Dialogues Clin Neurosci. 2017;19:259–69.
17. Phillips DM. JCAHO pain management standards are unveiled. Joint Commission on Accreditation of Healthcare Organizations. JAMA. 2000;284:428–9. https://doi.org/10.1001/jama.284.4.423b.
18. Farisco M, Evers K, Changeux JP. Drug addiction: from neuroscience to ethics. Front Psychiatry. 2018;9. https://www.frontiersin.org/articles/10.3389/fpsyt.2018.00595. https://doi.org/10.3389/fpsyt.2018.005.
19. Richardson L. Man faces felony charge in HIV case. New York Times, August 20, 1998.
20. Reamer F. AIDS, social work, and the "duty to protect". Social Work. 1991;36(1):56–60.
21. National Association of Social Workers. Ethical issues, HIV/AIDS, and social work practice. Workshop sponsored by the HIV/AIDS Spectrum: Mental Health Training and Education of Social Workers Project, 1997.
22. Millard WB. Grounding frequent flyers, not abandoning them: drug seekers in the ED. Ann Emerg Med. 2007;49(4):482–6.
23. McCaffery M, Grimm M, Pasero C, et al. On the meaning of "drug seeking.". Pain Manag Nurs. 2005;6(4):122–36.
24. "Cases Against Doctors" web page, U.S. Drug Enforcement Agency Office of Diversion Control web site, Available at: http://www.deadiversion.usdoj.gov/crim_admin_actions/index.html. Accessed 9 Feb 2010.
25. Chou R, Gilbert FJ, Fine PG, et al. Opioids for chronic noncancer pain: prediction and identification of aberrant drug-related behaviors: a review of the evidence for an American Pain Society and American Academy of Pain Medicine clinical practice guideline. J Pain. 2009;10(2):131–46.
26. Opioid risk assessment tool (ORT) assessment instrument. Clinical Tools Inc.; 2015.
27. Nicolaidis C. Police officer, deal-maker, or health care provider? Moving to a patient-centered framework for chronic opioid management. Pain Med. 2011;12:890–7.
28. Holliday S, Hayes C, Dunlop A. Opioid use in chronic non-cancer pain – part 2: prescribing issues and alternatives. Aust Fam Physician. 2013;42:104–11.

Chapter 33
Models of Doctor–Patient Relationship

Certain aspects of the provider–patient relationship are widely acknowledged and generally uncontroversial. This relationship is regarded as fiduciary, built on a foundation of trust. Patients entrust their healthcare to the provider, who, in turn, is expected to fulfil specific duties toward the patient. These obligations include: Demonstrating technical competence in the provider's area of expertise; taking actions to avoid causing harm to the patient (non-maleficence); acting for the patient's benefit (beneficence); and maintaining confidentiality of patient information under normal circumstances [1].

In 1847, the American Medical Association's code of medical ethics it is written that "The life of a sick person can be shortened not only by the acts, but also by the words or the manner of a physician. It is, therefore, a sacred duty to guard himself carefully in this respect, and to avoid all things which have a tendency to discourage the patient and to depress his spirits [1, 2].

Furthermore, the provider is recognised as a professional, bound by standards and expectations that encompass established mastery of requisite skills, possession of authoritative knowledge, expectations of appropriate behaviour and judgment, high-quality performance, devotion to the area or field of expertise, and adherence to codes of ethical conduct.

From the 1970s onward, there was a significant shift in the doctor-patient dynamic, marked by a heightened acknowledgment of the crucial role of patient autonomy in the decision-making process. In 1992 Emanuel et had defined four models of the relationship that characterise the physician–patient relationship.

1. Paternalistic model: The paternalistic model is a traditional approach, a *priestly,* where the doctor takes on a paternal role, making decisions on behalf of the patient without necessarily involving them in the decision-making process. The priestly model dates back to the Hippocratic tradition: "I will use treatment to help the sick according to my ability and *judgment*, but I will never use it to injure or wrong them". Priestly physician operates on the *medical model*, which treats patients as illnesses, not as persons. In this model, the doctor assumes the

S. Abbas, *Medical Ethics*, https://doi.org/10.1007/978-981-96-9199-9_33

role of an authoritative figure who acts in the best interest of the patient, often based on their own judgment and medical expertise. The patient may have limited involvement in the decision-making process, and the doctor may not fully discuss treatment options or consider the patient's preferences. The paternalistic model has been criticised for potentially disregarding patient autonomy and preferences, and it may not align with the principles of informed consent and respect for individual values that are emphasised in modern medical ethics. The modern healthcare systems encourage a more collaborative approach, where doctors and patients work together to make decisions that consider the patient's values, preferences. Paternalism extends beyond the realm of healthcare and is evident in familial dynamics. Common parental choices within a family exhibit paternalistic tendencies, where parents selectively share information with their children, present only favoured options, and take charge of significant decisions. Similarly, governmental mandates, such as requiring seatbelt or motorcycle helmet use, reflect a paternalistic approach. In these instances, the government asserts that it acts in the citizens' best interests, yet the paternalistic nature lies in the limitation of individual freedom to make those decisions without violating the law. One prevalent justification for paternalism in healthcare revolves around the notion that professionals, due to their significantly superior technical expertise and medical knowledge make this more logical for the provider, armed with this specialised knowledge, to assess the available options and make decisions. The rationale behind this perspective is that patients, often grappling with the complexities of technical details, may find themselves overwhelmed and, consequently, are not ideally positioned to make informed decisions. Moreover, individuals suffering from illnesses are frequently in a weakened and vulnerable state, turning to healthcare providers for expert advice, assistance, and judgment that may surpass the patient's own capacity [2, 3].

2. Informative Model

   Also referred to as the scientific, or consumer model. In this approach to the physician-patient interaction, the primary goal is for the physician to furnish the patient with all pertinent information. The patient, in turn, is expected to choose the medical interventions they desire, with the physician then executing the selected interventions. Within this model, the physician educates the patient on their disease state, potential diagnostic and therapeutic interventions, the nature and likelihood of associated risks and benefits, and any existing uncertainties in knowledge. At its extreme, patients could become acquainted with all medical information relevant to their condition, making choices based on interventions that best align with their values.

   The informative model operates under the assumption of a clear distinction between facts and values. The patient's values are presumed to be well-defined and known, with the patient primarily lacking factual information. In this model, there is an understanding of the patient's values and their judgment. The role of the physician in the informative model is that of a *technical expert*, offering the patient the tools to exercise control. As technical experts, physicians have significant responsibilities, including providing truthful information, maintaining competence in their area of expertise, and seeking consultation when their knowledge or skills are insufficient. The concept of patient autonomy is central to this model with a focus on patient's control over decision-making [2, 3].

3. Deliberative Model: Where the physician–patient interaction aims to assist the patient in determining and choosing the most suitable health-related values applicable to the clinical situation. The physician is tasked with providing information about the patient's clinical condition and aiding in the clarification of values inherent in the available options. The physician's goals encompass suggesting why certain health-related values are deemed more commendable in particular situations. Furthermore, the physician seeks no more than moral persuasion, avoiding coercion, and leaving the patient to define their life and select the values to be embraced.

   In the deliberative model, the physician assumes a role akin to a *teacher or friend.* Beyond merely indicating what the patient could do, the physician, acquainted with the patient's well-being and desiring what is best, suggests what the patient should do, outlining an admirable decision regarding medical therapy. The concept of patient autonomy in the deliberative model revolves around moral self-development, empowering the patient to contemplate, through dialogue, alternative health-related values, their worth, and their implications for treatment [3, 4].

4. The Interpretive Model: The interpretive model, aims to clarify the patient's values, assisting them in selecting medical interventions that align with these values. Similar to the informative model, the interpretive physician provides information about the condition, as well as the risks and benefits of potential interventions. However, the interpretive physician goes beyond this by helping the patient articulate their values and determining which medical interventions best align with these, essentially interpreting the patient's values for them.

In the interpretive model, the patient's values may not be fixed or fully known to the patient; they could be unclear or conflicting when applied to specific situations. Therefore, the physician collaborates with the patient to elucidate and make coherent these values. This involves working together to reconstruct the patient's goals, aspirations, commitments, and character. Importantly, the physician doesn't impose decisions on the patient; the ultimate choice lies with the patient, who decides which values and course of action best align with their identity. The physician assists the patient in understanding and applying their values without judgment.

In the interpretive model, the physician serves as a counsellor, akin to an advisory role. This involves supplying relevant information, aiding in clarifying values, and suggesting medical interventions that realise these values. Therefore, the physician's responsibility is to provide information and engage the patient in a collaborative process of understanding. Consequently, the concept of patient autonomy in the interpretive model centres around self-understanding; the patient gains clearer insight into who they are and how various medical options impact their identity.

The last two also used to be called the collaborative model. In the Collaborative Contractual Model, the physician and patient establish a mutually agreeable contract, resembling more of a biblical *covenant* than a legal construct.

The theoretical models of the doctor–patient relationship typically isolate the patient from their family and social context. However, in reality, patients often prefer not to make decisions in isolation. Many patients express a desire for the involvement of family or friends and seek advice from close relations, such as a spouse, son, or daughter, before arriving at a final decision. At times, they may even delegate decisions to individuals they believe possess better judgment or a more comprehensive understanding of the facts. The current model of a solitary, autonomous patient and a single physician in a decision-making context tends to overlook the preferences of such patients. In essence, there exists significant variability in patients' preferences for decision models, challenging the notion that a single, universal model can effectively cater to all individuals.

Given the diverse preferences regarding communication, it is unrealistic to assume that a single decision-making model would be suitable for all patients [4, 5].

Physicians can navigate in the right direction and consider individual patient differences effectively by initiating the process with a few straightforward questions: (1) How would you prefer communication and decision-making to be handled? (2) Who would you like to have present for support and advice when discussing treatment options with the physician? (3) How much information about the case would you like the doctor to share with you? and (4) In which of the numerous clinical decisions do you wish to participate? The responses to these questions would establish boundaries for the collaborative decision-making process within the patient's family and social context [3, 5].

References

1. Ezekiel J, Emanuel MD, Emanuel LL. The physician-patient relationship. JAMA. 1992;267(16):2221–6.
2. Clarke G, Hall RT, Rosencrance G. Physician-patient relations: no more models. Am J Bioeth. 2004;4(2):16–9.
3. Veach R. Models for ethical medicine in a revolutionary age. Hastings Center Report. 1972(June):2(3).
4. AMA Code of Ethics for Physicians, accessible at: https://www.ama-assn.org/sites/default/files/media-browser/principles-of-medical-ethics.pdf.
5. Pellegrino ED, Thomasma DC. For the Patient's Good: the Restoration of Beneficence in Health Care.

Chapter 34
Breaking Bad News

Hippocrates advise was "concealing most things from the patient while you are attending to him. Give necessary orders with cheerfulness and serenity…revealing nothing of the patient's future or present condition. For many patients…have taken a turn for the worse…by forecast of what is to come"

Breaking bad news is not a skill on its own, it is a type of communication. The concept of bad news, as defined, encapsulates information that significantly and adversely impacts an individual's perception of their future. This definition implies that bad news goes beyond merely conveying negative information; it goes to the core of an individual's outlook and expectations for what lies ahead. Bad news has the power to disrupt and reshape one's perspective on life, creating a profound emotional and psychological impact.

The severity of bad news is characterised by its potential to alter the course of an individual's life, introducing challenges or changes that may be unexpected and unwelcome. It is not just about the immediate negative implications; rather, it extends to how this information can shape an individual's long-term aspirations, plans, and sense of well-being.

The bad news is not limited to terminal cancer, it can be encountered in various situation such as intrauterine death, a new diagnosis of multiple sclerosis, or the need for emergency surgery a day before an important social event or organised overseas trip.

Understanding bad news in this way emphasises the emotional and existential dimensions that such information carries. It underscores the need for empathy and support when delivering or receiving bad news, recognising that the impact goes beyond the immediate circumstances and extends into the individual's broader sense of self and their place in the world [1].

Delivering distressing information to cancer patients is inherently unpleasant, often likened to "striking the patient over the head" or "dropping a bombshell." [2].

Professional cyclist Lance Armstrong's, memory of receiving a diagnosis of metastatic testicular cancer illustrates how the delivery of distressing news can

S. Abbas, *Medical Ethics*, https://doi.org/10.1007/978-981-96-9199-9_34

profoundly affect one's self-image "I left my house on October 2, 1996, as one person and came home another" [3].

The conveyer of negative information frequently undergoes intense emotions, including anxiety, a sense of responsibility, and a fear of facing negative judgment. This emotional strain leads to a hesitation in delivering bad news, a phenomenon termed the "MUM" effect. The impact of the MUM effect is notably pronounced when the recipient of the unfortunate news is already perceived as being in a distressed state [4].

When physicians feel uneasy about delivering bad news, they might sidestep discussions involving distressing information, trying not to take away hope, such as a grim prognosis, and unintentionally present an overly optimistic outlook to the patient. They might be worried about patient emotional reaction and don't know how to deal with it. Establishing a plan to ascertain the patient's values, preferences for involvement in decision-making, and a method for addressing their distress during the disclosure of unfavourable medical information can enhance a physician's confidence in handling such challenging conversations [5].

The act of sharing unfavourable information is an effort to accomplish four crucial objectives. Initially, it involves

1. Gathering information from the patient, enables the physician to gauge the patient's existing knowledge, expectations, and preparedness for receiving the distressing news.
2. Deliver clear and relevant information aligned with the patient's preferences and requirements.
3. Provide support to the patient by employing techniques that alleviate the emotional impact and sense of isolation often felt by those receiving bad news.
4. Strategy, typically in the form of a treatment plan, collaboratively with the patient's input.

It is easier to break task into a series of small tasks preceded by mental rehearsal of the tasks. The acronym SPIKES developed by Walter Baile and colleagues at the University of Texas MD Anderson Cancer Centre, stands for Setting up, Perception, Invitation, Knowledge, Emotions with Empathy, and Strategy or Summary.

1. Setting: setting should be conducive to undistracted and focused discussion for which privacy is essential. Patients are encouraged to bring significant others, ideally two, it is also important to remove barriers between you and the patient in a meeting where everyone is sitting. Eye contact brings connection and builds rapport with the patient, touching the patient on the arm or holding their hand is a good way to establish rapport. Allow generous time and avoid interruptions. If you have no experience then invite a senior colleague to do it and learn from them.
2. Perception of the situation regarding the illness or test results. Familiarise yourself with all the relevant clinical details and test results. At this step "ask before you tell." Employ open-ended questions to construct a reasonable understanding of how the patient interprets their medical situation—identifying its nature and assessing its perceived severity. Such as "What do you know about your

condition, or what have you been told about your condition." Additionally, it can help to discern whether the patient is experiencing any form of illness denial, such as wishful thinking, omitting crucial but unfavourable medical details, or harbouring unrealistic expectations of treatment [6].

3. Obtaining patient's Invitation: Discussing information disclosure can prompt the physician to plan the subsequent patient discussion. Ask about the patient's preferences for receiving test results—whether they want comprehensive information or a summary with more focus on the treatment plan. If patients prefer limited details, offer to address future questions or involve a relative or friend in the discussion [1, 7].
4. Knowledge of the medical facts and their implication before initiating the conversation. Warn the patient that bad news is coming, and that will reduce the impact of the bad news; you could say "I'm sorry but it is not looking good, or unfortunately I have bad news to tell you." Tailor your discussion to the patient's comprehension and vocabulary. Opt for nontechnical terms like "spread" instead of "metastasized." Refrain from excessive bluntness, as overly stark statements may lead to patient isolation and resentment. Provide information in manageable portions, periodically checking the patient's understanding. Refrain from engaging in arguments or criticism with colleagues and avoid becoming defensive about your own or a colleague's medical care. When the prognosis is bleak, avoid phrases like "There is nothing more we can do for you," recognising that patients often have other important goals such as symptom relief or end-of-life care [8, 9].
5. Empathy: explore the emotions raised during the interview. It is notoriously challenging to respond to a patient's emotions, which vary from denial, shock, crying, silence, or anger. Usually, the emotional reaction is expressed as shock, isolation, and grief. At this step physician needs to observe those emotions; name the emotion for what you thinks it is to oneself; identify the reason for such emotional reaction, ask the patient if in doubt. After allowing the patient a brief moment to express their feelings, inform them that you have identified the emotion and its underlying cause by providing a connecting statement [10]. An example is a 64-year-old woman who sees her medical oncologist after finishing six cycles of neo-adjuvant chemotherapy for pancreatic cancer; "I am sorry I have bad news: the chemo is not working, unfortunately the cancer grown somewhat. The patient starts to cry, the doctor offers tissue, moves his chair closer and hold the patient's hand, "I wish I have better news for you," be aware of cultural differences, some people don't like being touched. Doctor would pause here and allow the patient to express her emotions and regain her exposure" [1]. The doctor would express their own sadness or their worries. Assure the patient that you will be available when they need you and schedule a follow-up appointment (Table 34.1).
6. Establish a Strategy for Management:
   Conveying available treatment options to patients is not only a legal requirement in certain cases but also fosters the perception that the physician values their preferences. Having a clear plan for the future can significantly impact a patient's

Table 34.1 Examples of empathic, exploratory, and validating responses

Empathic statements	Exploratory questions	Validating responses
"I can see how upsetting this is to you."	"How do you mean?"	"I can understand how you felt that way."
"I can tell you weren't expecting to hear this."	"Tell me more about it."	"I guess anyone might have that same reaction."
"I know this is not good news for you."	"Could you explain what you mean?"	"You were perfectly correct to think that way."
"I'm sorry to have to tell you this."	"You said it frightened you?"	"Yes, your understanding of the reason for the tests is very good."
"This is very difficult for me also."	"Could you tell me what you're worried about?"	"It appears that you've thought things through very well."
"I was also hoping for a better result."	"Now, you said you were concerned about your children. Tell me more."	"Many other patients have had a similar experience."

emotional well-being and reduce feelings of anxiety and uncertainty. When individuals are aware of the steps, strategies, or courses of action they need to take, it provides a sense of structure and direction. This clarity in planning can offer several benefits:

Sense of control reduced Anxiety. Increased confidence, and better adherence to treatment. Patients with a clear plan are more likely to adhere to prescribed treatments and follow medical recommendations. Understanding the rationale behind each step fosters a commitment to the process, leading to improved health outcomes.

In essence, a clear plan for the future empowers patients to actively engage in their healthcare journey. It provides a roadmap that not only addresses the immediate concerns but also instills a sense of purpose, direction, and confidence in facing the challenges ahead. Healthcare providers play a crucial role in collaboratively developing and communicating these plans, ensuring that patients feel supported, informed, and in control of their health trajectory [11].

In the aftermath of traumatic deaths, individuals who have lost family members often place significant emphasis on specific aspects of how bad news is delivered. The perceived importance lies in the demeanour or attitude of the person delivering the news, the clarity with which the message is conveyed, the degree of privacy afforded during the disclosure, and the ability of the person delivering the news to effectively address questions.

1. Attitude of the Person Giving the News
   The emotional and empathetic approach of the individual delivering the news plays a pivotal role. A compassionate and supportive demeanour can contribute to a sense of understanding and shared grief, helping to ease the emotional impact on grieving family members.
2. Clarity of the Message
   The clear and straightforward communication of the information is crucial. Ambiguity or unclear messaging can lead to confusion and increased distress.

Providing a transparent account of the situation helps family members comprehend the gravity of the news and navigate the subsequent emotions more effectively.

3. Privacy During the Disclosure
   Privacy is considered a fundamental aspect of delivering bad news. Creating a private and quiet space for disclosure allows family members to process the information without the added stress of external distractions. It fosters an environment where individuals can react to the news more authentically and openly express their emotions.
4. Ability to Answer Questions
   The capability of the person delivering the news to address questions and concerns is highly valued. It demonstrates a readiness to provide support and information, helping family members make sense of the situation and aiding in the initial stages of coping with the loss.

References

1. Buckman R. Breaking bad news: a guide for health care professionals. Baltimore: Johns Hopkins University Press; 1992. p. 15.
2. Armstrong L. It's not about the bike: my journey back to life. New York: Putnam; 2000.
3. Miyaji N. The power of compassion: truth-telling among American doctors in the care of dying patients. Soc Sci Med. 1993;36:249–64.
4. Tesser, Conlee MC. Recipient emotionality as a determinant of the transmission of bad news. Proc Annu Conv Am Psych Assoc. 1973:247–8.
5. Baile WF, Lenzi R, Kudelka AP, et al. Improving physician-patient communication in cancer care: outcome of a workshop for oncologists. J Cancer Educ. 1997;12:166–73.
6. Lubinsky MS. Bearing bad news: dealing with the mimics of denial. Genet Couns. 1999;3:5–12.
7. Conlee MC, Tesser A. The effects of recipient desire to hear on news transmission. Sociometry. 1973;36:588–99.
8. Greisinger AJ, Lorimor RJ, Aday LA, et al. Terminally ill cancer patients: their most important concerns. Cancer Pract. 1997;5:147–54.
9. Maynard DW. On “realization” in everyday life: the forecasting of bad news as a social relation. Am Sociol Rev. 1996;61:109–31.
10. Ptacek JT, Eberhardt TL. Breaking bad news. A review of the literature. JAMA. 1996;276:496–502.
11. Nattinger, Hoffman RG, Sharpiro R, et al. The effects of legislative requirements on the use of breast conserving surgery. N Engl J Med. 1996;335:1035–40.

Chapter 35
Artificial Intelligence

AI in medicine is not new It is been developing since the 1950s and 1960s when early computers started aiding medical diagnosis and decision-making. AI systems in medicine started in the 1950s and continued through the 1980s The first AI programs were rule-based systems for diagnosis and treatment. MYCIN, developed in the 1970s at Stanford University, helped diagnose bacterial infections and suggest antibiotics. It was one of the first expert systems in medicine, using rule-based logic to analyse patient data and recommend antibiotics.

However, these systems used fixed rules and could not adapt to new medical info. As computing power grew AI moved from rule-based systems to machine learning letting models learn from medical data. IBM Watson Health, launched in 2011, draws attention to processing extensive medical literature and aiding to personalise oncology treatments. Watson helped pharmaceutical companies like *Pfizer* analyse biomedical data to identify potential drug candidates faster. The implementation of modern AI in medicine could revolutionise clinical decision-making. Ethical artificial intelligence implementation should meticulously focus on enhancing human expertise rather than merely supplanting it.

Deep learning and neural networks transformed AI in medicine. AI systems like Google's DeepMind Health are highly accurate in diagnosing eye diseases and predicting kidney failure and have been involved in developing tools for early cancer detection.

AI is used in personalised medicine, robotic surgery, virtual health helpers, and finding new drugs. Also, it boosts telemedicine, predicts disease outbreaks, and streamlines hospital tasks. Regulatory bodies such as the FDA now approve AI diagnostic tools for use. Ethical and bias issues persist [1–3].

Healthcare systems around the world are dealing with higher costs and worse results. This is a very tough problem to solve because it has many causes and is hard to understand. To fix it, many people, including those who make laws, doctors, and computer experts, think that using artificial intelligence (AI) could help to solve some of these problems [4].

S. Abbas, *Medical Ethics*, https://doi.org/10.1007/978-981-96-9199-9_35

Large language models (LLMs) are part of generative AI (GenAI), which creates natural language. This ability to mimic human communication brings ethical challenges like misinformation, trust issues, manipulation, and over-reliance on AI content. Careful ethical oversight and responsible development are crucial.

If harnessed with meticulous care, the collaboration between AI and clinicians, wherein AI delivers exhaustive, evidence-based clinical decision support to healthcare professionals (AI-Health), could present substantial opportunities for enhancing healthcare services and, ultimately, the well-being of patients [4].

New tech raises concerns that it may introduce errors and data breaches In healthcare, mistakes can severely harm patients especially when they are most vulnerable.

The Collingridge dilemma is especially pertinent to Artificial Intelligence (AI) in healthcare:

During the nascent stages of AI development: When AI is still in its formative phases, it is challenging to anticipate the full spectrum of ethical, safety, and social ramifications.

Upon widespread AI integration: Once AI is profoundly embedded in healthcare systems, instituting significant regulatory reforms or ethical adjustments becomes considerably more arduous.

This conundrum highlights the imperative for proactive and adaptable regulation, ensuring that AI and other nascent technologies advance responsibly while mitigating unforeseen repercussions [5].

Unleashing the full potential of artificial intelligence in healthcare necessitates tackling four crucial ethical quandaries: securing informed consent for data utilisation; guaranteeing safety and transparency; ensuring algorithmic fairness and minimising bias; and safeguarding data privacy. Each of these elements is intricately woven into the fabric of maintaining AI-driven healthcare as both ethical and efficacious [6].

The use of AI in healthcare raises concerns about accountability, as it may become unclear who is responsible for any harm caused. With the full extent of potential risks still unknown, which may significantly limit our ability to assign blame and ensure responsibility [7].

One of the inherent problems with AI is its complexity which makes it difficult to understand how the algorithms were developed, the fact they are difficult for non-experts to interpret, and the confusion that follows [8].

It is critical to minimise bias in the development of algorithms of AI in healthcare system to ensure communal fairness which requires diversification of data that is used in high-quality datasets to reduce the impact that the models may have on minorities. It also requires adequate transparency so doctors can justify AI-assisted decisions [9].

Governments and healthcare-institutions must establish lucid and stringent oversight and regulations for the utilisation of AI in medicine. Without meticulous oversight, AI might be implemented in manners that inappropriately prioritise financial gain over the welfare of patients [10].

The growing reliance on AI in healthcare threatens to weaken essential human aspects of the doctor-patient relationship, including empathy, trust, and personalised care—all of which are vital for effective treatment and recovery. As AI systems increasingly assist with diagnostics, decision-making, and patient management, it is crucial to develop technologies that complement rather than replace human interaction. Ongoing research should focus on integrating AI in ways that enhance compassionate care, ensuring that technological progress does not come at the expense of meaningful doctor-patient connections [11].

References

1. Miller DD, Brown EW. Artificial intelligence in medical practice: the question to the answer? Am J Med. 2018;131:129–33.
2. De Fauw J, Ledsam JR, Romera-Paredes B, Nikolov S, Tomasev N, Blackwell S, et al. Clinically applicable deep learning for diagnosis and referral in retinal disease. Nat Med. 2018;24:1342–50.
3. Char DS, Abràmoff MD, Feudtner C. Identifying ethical considerations for machine learning healthcare applications. Am J Bioeth. 2020;20:7–17.
4. Morley J, Floridi L. An ethically mindful approach to AI for health care. SSRN Electron J. 2020;395:254–5.
5. Genus A, Stirling A. Collingridge and the dilemma of control: towards responsible and accountable innovation. Res Policy. 2018;47:61–9.
6. Gerke S, Minssen T, Cohen G. Ethical and legal challenges of artificial intelligence-driven healthcare. Artif Intell Healthcare. 2020:295–336.
7. Tigard DW. There is no techno-responsibility gap. Philos Technol. 2020;34:589–607.
8. Burrell J. How the machine "thinks": understanding opacity in machine learning algorithms. Big Data Soc. 2016:3.
9. Chen RJ, Wang JJ, Williamson DFK, Chen TY, Lipkova J, Lu MY, Sahai S, Mahmood F. Algorithmic fairness in artificial intelligence for medicine and healthcare. Nat Biomed Eng. 2023;7(6):719–42.
10. Mennella C, Maniscalco U, De Pietro G, Esposito M. Ethical and regulatory challenges of AI technologies in healthcare: a narrative review. Heliyon. 2024;10(4).
11. Akingbola A, Adeleke O, Idris A, Adewole O, Adegbesan A. Artificial intelligence and the dehumanization of patient care. J Med Surg Public Health. 2024;3:100138, SSN 2949-916X, https://doi.org/10.1016/j.glmedi.2024.100138.

MIX
Papier aus verantwortungsvollen Quellen
Paper from responsible sources
FSC® C105338

If you have any concerns about our products,
you can contact us on
ProductSafety@springernature.com

In case Publisher is established outside the EU,
the EU authorized representative is:
Springer Nature Customer Service Center GmbH
Europaplatz 3, 69115 Heidelberg, Germany

Printed by Libri Plureos GmbH
in Hamburg, Germany